W9-BIB-391

The Home Health Aide Handbook

Jetta Fuzy, RN, MS
William Leahy, MD

THIRD EDITION

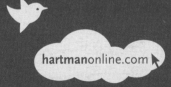

hartmanonline.com

Hartman

Acknowledgments

Managing Editor
Susan Hedman

Designer
Kirsten Browne

Production
Thad Castillo

Photography
Art Clifton/Dick Ruddy/Pat Berrett

Proofreader
Kristin Cartwright

Sales/Marketing
Debbie Rinker/Kendra Robertson/Erika Walker/Belinda Midyette

Customer Service
Fran Desmond/Thomas Noble/Angela Storey/Cheryl Garcia/Eliza Martin

Warehouse Coordinator
C.R. Beck

Special Thanks

A very warm thank-you goes to our insightful reviewer, Sally Lyle, RN, BSN, for her valuable suggestions.

Copyright Information

Notice to Readers

Though the guidelines and procedures contained in this text are based on consultations with healthcare professionals, they should not be considered absolute recommendations. The instructor and readers should follow employer, local, state, and federal guidelines concerning healthcare practices. These guidelines change, and it is the reader's responsibility to be aware of these changes and of the policies and procedures of his or her healthcare agency.

The publisher, author, editors, and reviewers cannot accept any responsibility for errors or omissions or for any consequences from application of the information in this book and make no warranty, expressed or implied, with respect to the contents of the book. The publisher does not warrant or guarantee any of the products described herein or perform any analysis in connection with any of the product information contained herein.

Gender Usage

This textbook utilizes the pronouns "he," "his," "she," and "hers" interchangeably to denote care team members and clients.

Contents

Procedure	Page	Procedure	Page

Procedures

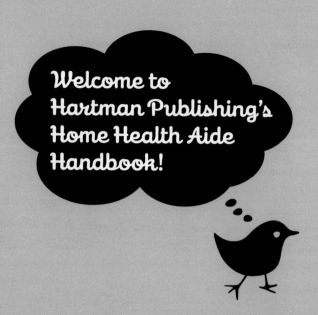

Welcome to
Hartman Publishing's
Home Health Aide
Handbook!

We hope you will happily place this little reference book into your purse, backpack, or your home care visit bag and leave it there so you will have it available at all times as you go about your day-to-day duties as a home health aide. This handbook will serve as a quick but comprehensive reference tool for you to use from client to client.

Features and Benefits

This book is a valuable tool for many reasons. For home health aides, it includes all the procedures you learned in your training program, plus references to abbreviations, medical terms, care guidelines for specific diseases, and an appendix for you to write down important names and phone numbers. For certified nursing assistants moving to home care, we've included information on making the transition from facilities to homes. In addition, this book contains all of the federal requirements for home health aides, so it can also be used in a basic training program.

We have divided the book into eight parts and assigned each part its own colored tab, which you'll see at the top of every page.

> I. Defining Home Health Services
>
> II. Foundation of Client Care
>
> III. Understanding Your Clients
>
> IV. Client Care
>
> V. Special Clients, Special Needs
>
> VI. Home Management and Nutrition
>
> VII. Caring for Yourself
>
> VIII. Appendix

You'll find **key terms** throughout the text. Explanations for these terms are in the Glossary in the Appendix of this book. Common Disorders, Guidelines and Observing and Reporting are also colored for easy reference. Procedures are indicated with a black bar. There is also an index in the back of the book. We will be updating this guide periodically, so don't hesitate to let us know what you would like to see in the next handbook we publish.

CONTACT US AT:
Hartman Publishing, Inc.,
8529 Indian School Rd NE
Albuquerque, NM 87112
Phone: (505) 291-1274
Fax: (505) 291-1284
Web: hartmanonline.com
E-mail: orders@hartmanonline.com

I.
Defining Home Health Services

Home Health Care

Home health aides provide assistance to the chronically ill, the elderly, and family caregivers who need relief from the stress of caregiving. Many home health aides also work in assisted living facilities, which provide independent living in a homelike group environment, with professional care available as needed. As advances in medicine and technology extend the lives of people with **chronic** illnesses, the number of people needing health care will increase. The need for home health aides will also increase.

Payers

Agencies pay you from payments they receive from the following payers:
- Insurance companies
- Health maintenance organizations **(HMO)**
- Preferred provider organizations **(PPO)**
- **Medicare**
- **Medicaid**
- Individual clients or family members

The Centers for Medicare & Medicaid Services (CMS), formerly the Health Care Finance Administration (HCFA), is a federal agency within the U.S. Department of Health and Human Services. CMS runs the Medicare and Medicaid programs at the federal level.

Medicare pays agencies a fixed fee for a 60-day period of care based on a client's condition. If the cost of providing care exceeds the payment, the agency loses money. If the care provided costs less than the payment, the agency makes money. For these reasons, home health agencies must pay close attention to costs. And because all payers monitor the quality of care provided, the way in which work is documented is very important.

CMS's payment system for home care is called the "home health prospective payment system" or "HH PPS."

Purpose of Home Care

Perhaps the most important reason for health care in the home is that most people who are ill or disabled feel more comfortable at home. Health care in familiar surroundings improves mental and physical well-being. It has proven to be a major factor in the healing process.

Agency Structure

Clients who need home care are referred to a home health agency by their doctors. They can also be referred by a hospital discharge planner, a social services agency, the state or local department of public health, the welfare office, a local Agency on Aging, or a senior center. Clients and family members can also choose an agency that meets their needs. Once an agency is chosen and the doctor has made a referral, a staff member performs an assessment of the client. This determines how the care needs can best be met. The home environment will also be evaluated to determine whether or not it is safe for the client.

Home health agencies employ many home health aides (HHAs) and certified nursing assistants (CNAs). Services provided may include nursing care, specialized therapy, specific medical equipment, nutrition therapy/dietary counseling, pharmacy and intravenous (IV) products, and personal care. The services provided depend on the size of the agency. Small agencies may provide basic nursing care, personal care, and housekeeping services. Larger agencies may provide speech, physical, and occupational therapies and medical social work. All home health agencies have professional staff who make decisions about what care and services are needed (Fig. 1-1).

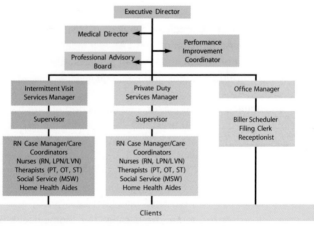

Fig. 1-1. *A typical home health agency organization chart.*

HHA's Role

A home health aide may be assigned to "make a visit." This means that he or she will spend a certain number of hours each day or week with a client to provide personal care and housekeeping services. While the supervisor or case manager develops the assignments and client care plans, input from all members of the care team is needed. All HHAs are under supervision of the skilled professional: a registered nurse, a physical therapist, or a speech therapist.

In some ways, working as a home health aide is similar to working as a nursing assistant. In addition to the basic medical procedures and many of the personal care procedures, your job will also include:

- **Housekeeping**: You may have housekeeping responsibilities, including cooking, cleaning, laundry, and grocery shopping, for at least some of your clients. Tasks must be prioritized according to the assignment description, the client's needs, and what time allows.

- **Family contact**: You may have a lot more contact with clients' families in the home than you would in a facility. You will work with the family as a team, encouraging them to participate as much as possible in meeting the goals of the care plan.

- **Independence**: You will work independently as a home health aide. Your supervisor will monitor your work, but you will spend most of your hours working with clients without direct supervision. Thus, you must be a responsible and independent worker.

- **Communication**: Communication skills are important. You must keep yourself informed of changes in the client care plan. You must also keep others informed of changes you observe in the client and the client's environment.

- **Transportation**: You will have to get yourself from one client's home to another. You will need to have a dependable car or know how to use public transportation. You may also face bad weather conditions. Clients need your care—rain, snow, or sleet.

- **Safety awareness**: You need to be aware of personal safety when you are traveling alone to visit clients. Be aware of your surroundings, walk confidently, and avoid dangerous situations, such as visits after dark.

- **Flexibility**: Each client's home will be different. You will need to adapt to the changes in environment. You will have to learn to work alone with only the client and family to help.

- **Adapting to the working environment**: In home care, the layout of rooms, stairs, lack of equipment, cramped bathrooms, rugs, clutter, and even pets can complicate caregiving.

- **Showing respect for the client's home**: In a client's home, you are a guest. You need to be respectful of the client's property and customs.

- **Providing comfort**: One of the best things about home care is that it allows clients to stay in the familiar and comfortable surroundings of their own homes.

As an HHA, you will be part of a team of health professionals that includes doctors, nurses, social workers, therapists, and specialists. The client and client's family are considered part of the team. Everyone involved will work closely together to help clients recover from illnesses or injuries. If full recovery is not possible, the team will help clients do as much as they can for themselves.

The Care Team

Clients will have different needs and problems. Healthcare professionals with different kinds of education and experience will help care for them. Members of the healthcare team may include:

Home Health Aide (HHA): The home health aide performs assigned tasks, such as taking vital signs, and provides routine personal care, such as bathing clients or preparing meals. HHAs spend more time with clients than other care team members do. That is why they act as the "eyes and ears" of the team. Observing and reporting changes in the client's condition or abilities is a very important duty of the HHA.

Case Manager or Supervisor: Usually a registered nurse, a case manager or a supervisor is assigned to each client by the home health agency. The case manager or supervisor, with input from other team members, creates the basic care plan for the client. He or she monitors any changes that are observed and reported by the HHA. The case manager also makes changes in the client care plan when necessary.

Registered Nurse (RN): In a home health agency, a registered nurse coordinates, manages, and provides care. RNs also supervise and train HHAs. They develop the HHA's assignments.

Doctor (MD or DO): A doctor's job is to diagnose disease or disability and prescribe treatment. A doctor generally decides when patients need home health care and refers them to home health agencies.

Physical Therapist (PT): A physical therapist evaluates a person and develops a treatment plan. Goals are to increase movement, improve circulation, promote healing, reduce pain, prevent disability, and regain or maintain mobility. A PT gives therapy in the form of heat, cold, massage, ultrasound, electricity, and exercise to muscles, bones, and joints.

Occupational Therapist (OT): An occupational therapist helps clients learn to compensate for disabilities. For clients in home care, an OT may help clients perform activities of daily living (ADLs), such as dressing, eating, and bathing.

Speech-Language Pathologist (SLP): A speech-language pathologist, or speech therapist, helps with speech and swallowing problems. An SLP identifies communication disorders, addresses factors involved in recovery, and develops a plan of care to meet recovery goals. An SLP teaches exercises that help the client improve or overcome speech problems. An SLP also evaluates a person's ability to swallow food and drink.

Registered Dietitian (RD): A registered dietitian teaches clients and their families about special diets to improve their health and help them manage their illness. RDs may supervise the preparation and service of food and educate others about healthy nutritional habits.

Medical Social Worker (MSW): A medical social worker determines clients' needs and helps them get support services, such as counseling, meal services, and financial assistance.

Client: The client is an important member of the care team. The client has the right to make decisions and choices about his or her own care. The client's family may also be involved in these decisions. The care team revolves around the client and his or her condition, treatment, and progress. Without the client, there is no care team.

The Care Plan

The care plan is individualized for each client. It is developed to help achieve the goals of care (Fig. 1-2). It lists tasks that team members, including home health aides, must perform. It states how often these tasks should be done and how they should be carried out.

The care plan is a guide to help the client attain and maintain the best level of health possible. **Activities not listed on the care plan should not be performed**. The HHA care plan is part of the overall plan of care. It must be followed very carefully.

Care planning should involve input from the client and/or the family, as well as health professionals. Professionals will assess the client's physical, financial, social, and psychological needs. After the doctor prescribes treatment, the supervisor, nurses, and other care team members create the care plan. Many factors are considered when creating the care plan. They include the client's health and physical condition, diagnosis, treatment, any additional services needed, and the client's home and family.

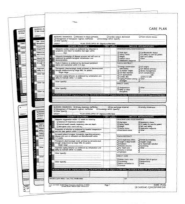

Fig. 1-2. *A sample client care plan.* (REPRINTED WITH PERMISSION OF BRIGGS COR- PORATION, DES MOINES, IOWA, 800-247-2343, WWW.BRIGGSCORP.COM)

Multiple care plans may be necessary for some clients. In these situations, the supervisor will coordinate the client's overall care. There will be one care plan for the HHA to follow. There will be separate care plans for other providers, such as the physical therapist.

Care plans must be updated as the client's condition changes. Reporting changes and problems to the supervisor is a very important duty of the home health aide. This allows the care team to revise care plans to meet the client's changing needs.

Chain of Command

As a home health aide, you are carrying out instructions given to you by a nurse. The nurse is acting on the instructions of a doctor or other member of the care team. This chain of command describes the line of authority and helps to make sure that your clients get proper care. It also protects you and your employer from liability. **Liability** is a legal term that means someone can be held responsible for harming someone else. For example, imagine that something you do for a client harms him. However, what you did was in the care plan and was done according to policy and procedure. Then you may not be liable, or responsible, for hurting the client. However, if you do something not in the care plan that harms a client, you could be held responsible. That is why it is important to follow instructions in the care plan and for the agency to have a chain of command (Fig. 1-3).

Home health aides must understand what they can and cannot do. This is important so that you do not harm a client or involve yourself or your employer in a lawsuit. Some states certify that a home health aide is qualified to work. However, home health aides are not licensed healthcare providers. Everything you do in your job is assigned to you by a licensed healthcare professional. You do your job under the authority of another person's license. That is why these professionals will show great interest in what you do and how you do it.

Every state grants the right to practice various jobs in health care through licensure. Examples include granting a license to practice nursing, medicine, or physical therapy. All members of the care team work under each professional's scope of practice. A **scope of practice** defines the things you are allowed to do and describes how to do them correctly.

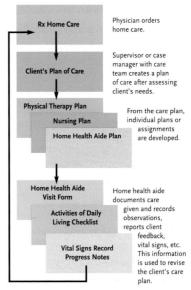

Fig. 1-3. *The chain of command describes the line of authority and helps ensure that the client receives proper care.*

Policies and Procedures

You will be told where to locate a list of policies and procedures that all staff members are expected to follow. A **policy** is a course of action that should be taken every time a certain situation occurs. For example, one policy at most agencies is that the care plan must be followed. That means that every time you visit a client, what you do will be determined by the care plan. A **procedure** is a particular method, or way, of doing something. For example, your agency will have a procedure for reporting information about your clients. The procedure tells you what form you fill out, when and how often to fill it out, and to whom it is given.

Common policies and procedures at home health agencies include the following:

- Keep all information confidential.
- Follow the client's care plan. Do not perform any tasks that are not included in the care plan.
- Report to the supervisor at regular arranged times, and more often if necessary.

- Report important events or changes in clients and their families.
- Do not discuss personal problems with the client or the client's family.
- Be punctual and dependable. Employers expect this of all employees.
- Follow deadlines for documentation and paperwork.
- Provide all client care in a pleasant, professional manner.
- Do not give or accept gifts.

Your employer will have policies and procedures for every client care situation. Though written procedures may seem long and complicated, each step is important.

Professionalism

Professional means having to do with work or a job. The opposite of professional is personal, which refers to your life outside your job. This includes your family, friends, and home life. Professionalism is how you behave when you are on the job. It includes how you dress, the words you use, and the things you talk about. It also includes being on time, finishing assignments, and reporting to your supervisor. For an HHA, professionalism means participating in care planning, making important observations, and reporting accurately.

Following the policies and procedures of your agency is an important part of professionalism. Clients, coworkers, and supervisors respect employees who behave in a professional way. Professionalism will help you keep your job and may help you earn promotions and raises.

A professional relationship with a client includes:

- Maintaining a positive attitude
- Being cleanly and neatly dressed and groomed (Fig. 1-4)
- Arriving on time, doing tasks efficiently, and leaving on time
- Finishing an assignment
- Doing only the tasks assigned
- Keeping all clients' information confidential
- Speaking politely and cheerfully to the client, even if you are not in a good mood

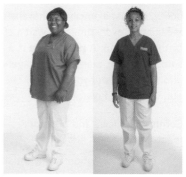

Fig. 1-4. *Good grooming includes being clean and neatly dressed. Keep long hair tied back, and wear clean clothes and comfortable, clean shoes.*

- Never cursing or using profanity, even if the client does
- Never discussing your personal problems
- Not giving or accepting gifts
- Calling the client "Mr.," "Mrs.," "Ms.," or "Miss," and his or her last name, or by the name he or she prefers
- Listening to the client
- Always explaining the care you will provide before providing it
- Always following care practices, such as handwashing, to protect yourself and the client

A professional relationship with an employer includes:

- Maintaining a positive attitude
- Completing assignments efficiently
- Consistently following policies and procedures
- Documenting and reporting carefully and correctly
- Communicating problems with clients or assignments
- Reporting anything that keeps you from completing assignments
- Asking questions when you do not know or understand something
- Taking directions or criticism without getting upset
- Always being on time
- Participating in education programs offered
- Being a positive role model for your agency at all times

Home health aides must be **compassionate**, honest, **tactful**, **conscientious**, dependable, respectful, unprejudiced, and tolerant.

Legal and Ethical Aspects

Ethics and laws guide our behavior. **Ethics** are the knowledge of right and wrong. An ethical person has a sense of duty toward others. He or she always tries to do what is right. If ethics tell us what we should do, **laws** tell us what we *must* do. Laws are rules set by the government to help people live peacefully together and to ensure order and safety.

Ethics and laws are very important in health care. They protect people receiving care and guide people giving care. Home health aides and all care team members should be guided by a code of ethics. They must know the laws that apply to their jobs.

Examples of legal and ethical behavior by HHAs include the following:

- Being honest at all times
- Protecting clients' privacy
- Not accepting gifts or tips
- Not becoming personally or sexually involved with clients or families
- Reporting abuse or suspected abuse of a client and assisting clients in reporting abuse if they wish to make a complaint of abuse
- Following the care plan and assignments
- Not performing any unassigned tasks or tasks outside their scope of practice
- Reporting all client observations and incidents
- Documenting accurately and promptly
- Following rules on safety and infection control, including OSHA rules about bloodborne pathogens, Standard Precautions, and tuberculosis

Clients' rights relate to how clients must be treated. They provide an ethical code of conduct for healthcare workers. Home health agencies give clients a list of these rights and review each right with them. Many states require home health agencies to provide their clients with the abuse hotline numbers. And it is a law for HHAs to report suspected cases of abuse.

Client's Bill of Rights

Home health clients and their formal caregivers have a right to not be discriminated against based on race, color, religion, national origin, age, sex, gender, sexual orientation, or disability. Furthermore, clients and caregivers have a right to mutual respect and dignity, including respect for property. Caregivers are prohibited from accepting personal gifts and borrowing from clients.

CLIENTS HAVE THE RIGHT:

- to have relationships with home health providers that are based on honesty and ethical standards of conduct;
- to be informed of the procedure they can follow to lodge complaints with the home health provider about the care that is, or fails to be, furnished and about a lack of respect for property [The phone number to report this listed here.];
- to know about the disposition of such complaints;
- to voice their grievances without fear of discrimination or reprisal for having done so; and
- to be advised of the telephone number and hours of operation of the state's home care hotline which receives questions and complaints about local home care agencies, including complaints about implementation of advance directive requirements. [Hours and phone number listed here.]

CLIENTS HAVE THE RIGHT:

- to be notified in advance about the care that is to be furnished, the disciplines of the caregivers who will furnish the care, and the frequency of the proposed visits;

- to be advised of any change in the plan of care before the change is made;

- to participate in planning care and planning changes in care, and to be advised that they have the right to do so;

- to be informed in writing of rights under state law to make decisions concerning medical care, including the right to accept or refuse treatment and the right to formulate advance directives;

- to be notified of the expected outcomes of care and any obstacles or barriers to treatment;*

- to be informed in writing of policies and procedures for implementing advance directives, including any limitations if the provider cannot implement an advance directive on the basis of conscience;

- to have healthcare providers comply with advance directives in accordance with state law;

- to receive care without condition or discrimination based on the execution of advance directives; and

- to refuse services without fear of reprisal or discrimination.

* The home care provider or the client's physician may be forced to refer the client to another source of care if the client's refusal to comply with the plan of care threatens to compromise the provider's commitment to quality care.

CLIENTS HAVE THE RIGHT:

- to confidentiality of the medical record as well as information about their health, social, and financial circumstances and about what takes place in the home; and

- to expect the home care provider to release information only as required by law or authorized by the client and to be informed of procedures for disclosure.

CLIENTS HAVE THE RIGHT:

- to be informed of the extent to which payment may be expected from Medicare, Medicaid, or any other payer known to the home care provider;

- to be informed of the charges that will not be covered by Medicare;

- to be informed of the charges for which the client may be liable;

- to receive this information orally and in writing before care is initiated and within 30 calendar days of the date the home care provider becomes aware of any changes; and

- to have access, upon request, to all bills for service the client has received regardless of whether the bills are paid out-of-pocket or by another party.

CLIENTS HAVE THE RIGHT:

- to receive care of the highest quality;

- in general, to be admitted by a home health provider only if it has the resources needed to provide the care safely and at the required level of intensity, as determined by a professional assessment; a provider with less than optimal resources may nevertheless admit the client if a more appropriate provider is not available, but only after fully informing the client of the provider's limitations and the lack of suitable alternative arrangements; and

- to be told what to do in the case of an emergency.

THE HOME HEALTH PROVIDER SHALL ASSURE THAT:

- all medically-related home care is provided in accordance with physicians' orders and that a plan of care specifies the services and their frequency and duration; and

- all medically-related personal care is provided by an appropriately trained home health aide who is supervised by a nurse or other qualified home care professional.

CLIENTS HAVE THE RESPONSIBILITY:

- to notify the provider of changes in their condition (e.g., hospitalization, changes in the plan of care, symptoms to be reported);

- to follow the plan of care;

- to notify the provider if the visit schedule needs to be changed;

- to inform providers of the existence of any changes made to advance directives;
- to advise the provider of any problems or dissatisfaction with the services provided;
- to provide a safe environment for care to be provided; and
- to carry out mutually-agreed-upon responsibilities.

To satisfy the Medicare certification requirements, the Centers for Medicare & Medicaid Services (CMS) requires that agencies:

1. Give a copy of the Bill of Rights to each client during the admission process.
2. Explain the Bill of Rights to the client and document that this has been done.

Agencies may have clients sign a copy of the Client's Bill of Rights to acknowledge receipt.

You can help protect your clients' rights in the following ways:

- Never **abuse** a client physically, **psychologically**, **verbally**, or **sexually**.
- Watch for and report to your supervisor any signs of abuse or **neglect**.
- Call the client by the name he or she prefers.
- Involve clients in your planning.
- Always explain a procedure before performing it.
- Respect a client's refusal of care. Report the refusal to your supervisor immediately.
- Tell your supervisor if a client has questions about the goals of care or the care plan.
- Be truthful when documenting care.
- Do not talk or gossip about a client.
- Knock and ask permission before entering a client's room.
- Do not open a client's mail or look through his belongings.
- Do not accept gifts or money from a client.
- Respect your clients' property.
- Report observations regarding a client's condition or care.

Observing and Reporting: Abuse and Neglect

O/R Physical abuse—unexplained injuries including burns, bruises, and bone injuries

O/R Psychological abuse—complaints of anxiety, signs of stress, withdrawal from others, or fear of family members, friends, or authority figures

O/R Neglect (**active** or **passive**)—signs of lack of care when HHA is not present, such as incontinence briefs not changed, or lack of food in the house

Negligence means actions, or the failure to act or provide the proper care for a client, that result in unintended injury. Some examples of negligence include:

- Not noticing that your client's dentures do not fit properly. Therefore, he is not eating well and becomes malnourished.

- Not replacing a hearing aid battery. Your client does not hear the smoke alarm, but is rescued by a neighbor who does hear it.

- Not observing that your client's eyesight is getting worse. Corrective measures are not taken, and she falls and is injured.

- Forgetting to lock a client's wheelchair before transferring her. The client falls and is injured.

To respect **confidentiality** means to keep private things private. You will learn confidential (private) information about your clients. You may learn about a client's state of health, finances, and personal relationships. Ethically and legally, you must protect the confidentiality of this information. This means you should not tell anyone other than members of the care team anything about your clients.

Congress passed the Health Insurance Portability and Accountability Act (HIPAA) in 1996. It was further defined and revised in 2001 and 2002. One of the reasons this law was passed is to help keep health information private and secure. All healthcare organizations must take special steps to protect health information. They and their employees can be fined and/or imprisoned if they do not follow special rules to protect privacy. This applies to all healthcare providers, including doctors, nurses, home health aides, and all care team members.

Under this law, health information must be kept private. It is called protected health information (PHI). Examples of PHI include name, address, telephone number, social security number, e-mail address, and medical record number. Only those who must have information to provide care or to process records should know this information. They must protect the information so it does not become known or used by anyone else. It must be kept confidential.

HHAs cannot give any information about a client to anyone who is not directly involved in the client's care unless the client gives official consent or unless the law requires it. For example, if a neighbor asks you how your client is doing, reply, "I'm sorry but I cannot share that information. It's confidential." That is the correct response to anyone who does not have a legal reason to know about the client.

All healthcare workers must follow HIPAA regulations, no matter where they are or what they are doing. There are serious penalties for violating these rules. Penalties differ depending upon the violation and can include fines and prison sentences.

Maintaining confidentiality is a legal and ethical obligation. It is part of respecting your clients and their rights. Discussing a client's care or personal affairs with anyone other than your supervisor or other members of the care team violates the law.

II.
Foundation of Client Care

Communication

Communication is the process of exchanging information with others. It is a process of sending and receiving messages. People communicate by using signs and symbols, such as words, drawings, and pictures. They also communicate by their behavior.

Effective communication is a critical part of your job. HHAs must communicate with supervisors, members of the care team, clients, and family members. A client's health depends on how well you communicate your observations and concerns to your supervisor. You will also need to be able to communicate clearly and respectfully in stressful or confusing situations.

Clients may sometimes display combative, meaning violent or hostile, behavior. Such behavior may include hitting, pushing, kicking, or verbal attacks. This behavior may be the result of disease affecting the brain. It may also be an expression of frustration. Or it may just be part of someone's personality. In general, combative behavior is not a reaction to you. Do not take it personally.

Always report combative behavior to your supervisor and document it. Even if you do not find the behavior upsetting, the care team needs to be aware of it. Some ways of coping with combative behavior include the following:

- Block physical blows or step out of the way, but never hit back.

- Leave the client alone if you can safely do so.

- Do not respond to verbal attacks.

- Consider what provoked the client.

- Report inappropriate behavior to your supervisor.

Barriers to Communication

Communication can be blocked or disrupted in many ways. Following are some barriers and ways to avoid them:

- Client does not hear you, does not hear correctly, or does not understand. Stand directly facing the client. Speak more slowly than you do with family and friends. Speak clearly, in a low, pleasant voice.

- Client is difficult to understand. Be patient and take time to listen. Ask client to repeat or explain. Rephrase the message in your own words to make sure you have understood.

- Message uses words receiver does not understand. Do not use medical terminology with clients. Speak in simple, everyday words. Ask what a word means if you are not sure.

- Using slang confuses the message. Avoid using slang words and expressions that are unprofessional or may not be understood. Do not use profanity, even if the client does.

- Avoid using clichés. Clichés are phrases that are used over and over again and don't really mean anything. For example, "Everything will be fine" is a cliché.

- Asking "Why?" makes the client defensive. Avoid asking "Why?" when a client makes a statement.

- Giving advice is inappropriate. Do not offer your personal opinion or give advice.

- Client may speak a different language. Speak slowly and clearly. Keep your messages short and simple. You may need to use pictures or gestures to communicate.

- **Nonverbal communication** changes the message. Be aware of your body language and gestures when you are speaking.

Oral Reports

Ask for more. When clients report symptoms, events, or feelings, have them repeat what they have said and ask them for more information. Avoid asking questions that can be easily answered with a simple "yes" or "no" response. Instead ask questions that encourage the client to offer more descriptive information. For example, asking the client, "Did you sleep well last night?" could easily be answered "yes" or "no." However, asking the client, "Tell me about your night and how you slept," is more likely to encourage the client to offer facts and details.

HHAs must be able to make brief and accurate oral and written presentations to clients and staff. Reports of a client's status are used in two ways. The first is to report something your supervisor needs to know about immediately. Signs and symptoms that should be reported will be discussed throughout this book. In addition, anything that endangers your client should be reported immediately. Examples include the following:

- Falls
- Chest pain
- Severe headache
- Difficulty breathing
- Abnormal pulse, respiration, or blood pressure
- Change in client's mental status
- Sudden weakness or loss of mobility
- High fever
- Loss of consciousness
- Change in level of consciousness
- Bleeding
- Change in client's condition
- Bruises, abrasions, or other signs of possible abuse

Another way to use oral reports is to discuss your experiences with a client or family member and your observations of the client's condition and care. These reports should be facts, not opinions. Even for oral reports, write notes so you do not forget any details. You will also have to make a written report later, so you will need to be able to recall all the facts accurately. Following an oral report, document when, why, about what, and to whom an oral report was given.

Sometimes your supervisor or another member of the care team will give you a brief oral report on one of your clients. Listen carefully and take notes if needed. Ask about anything you do not understand. At the end of the conversation, restate what you have been told to make sure you understand.

In order to report accurately, observe your clients, their families, and their homes. To observe accurately, use as many senses as possible to gather information. Some examples follow:

- **Sight**. Look for changes in client's appearance. These include rashes, redness, paleness, swelling, discharge, weakness, sunken eyes, and posture or gait (walking) changes. Look for changes in the home. Does the home appear disorganized or dirty? Is food needed? Do safety hazards exist?

- **Hearing.** Listen to what the client tells you about his or her condition, family, or needs. Is the client speaking clearly and making sense? Does the client show emotions such as anger, frustration, or sadness? Is breathing normal? Does client wheeze, gasp, or cough? Is the area calm and quiet enough for your client to rest as needed?

- **Touch.** Does your client's skin feel hot or cool, moist or dry? Is pulse rate normal? Use your sense of touch to test the bath water and the home's heating or cooling system.

- **Smell**. Do you notice odor from the client's body? Odors could suggest inadequate bathing, infections, or **incontinence**. Breath odor could suggest use of alcohol or tobacco, indigestion, or poor oral care. Odors in the home may suggest housecleaning or repairs are needed. Food odors could indicate spoilage.

Using all your senses will allow you to make the most complete report of a client's situation.

Documentation

Maintaining current documentation means keeping a record of everything you do and observe during a client visit. You and your agency maintain current documentation for these reasons:

1. It is the only way to guarantee clear and complete communication between all the members of the care team.

2. Documentation is a legal record of every part of a client's treatment. It is proof that a visit was actually made. Medical charts can be used in court as legal evidence.

3. Documentation protects you and your employer from liability by proving what you did on every visit with your client.

4. Documentation provides an up-to-date record of the status and care of each client.

Visit records, progress notes, or clinical notes are the notes you make each time you visit a client. These notes serve as a record of your visit and the care you provided. Visit records also document observations of the client's condition, change, or progress (improvement). When writing visit records, observe these rules:

- Write your notes immediately after the visit. This helps you remember important details. Always wait to document care until after you have completed it. Never record any care before it is done.

- Think about what you want to say before writing. Be as brief and as clear as possible.

- Write facts, not opinions. For example, "Client has lost 2 lbs. Did not finish lunch," reports facts. It is more useful than, "Client is thin and won't eat." When reporting something a client or family member told you, put the words in quotation marks (" "). Document the tasks that you performed, assisted with, or observed.

- Write as neatly as you can. Use black ink.

- If you make a mistake, draw one line through it. Write the correct word or words. Put your initials and the date. Never erase something you have written. Never use correction fluid (Fig. 2-1).

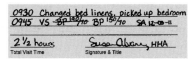

Fig. 2-1. *Corrected notes.*

- Sign your full name, write your title (Home Health Aide, Aide, or HHA). Write the date after each day's visit notes.

- Document as specified in the care plan. Some agencies have a "check-off" sheet for documenting care. It is also called an ADL (activities of daily living) sheet.

Incident reports must be completed when an accident or other significant event occurs during a visit. Report the incident as soon as possible. Report it before leaving the client's home. Always check with your supervisor before completing the report. Every home health agency has its own policies and procedures for incident reporting.

In general, file a report when any of the following incidents occur:

- Your client falls.

- You or a client breaks or damages something.

- Your client or a family member makes a request that is out of your scope of practice or not on your assignment sheet.

- Your client or a family member makes sexual advances or remarks.

- Anything happens that makes you feel uncomfortable, threatened, or unsafe.

- You get injured on the job.

- You are exposed to blood or body fluids.

An incident report documents events that happen in the home and protects you. It provides a written record of anything that happens and describes your part in it. Most agencies use incident reports in place of writing up the accident on the visit form. You may be asked to document that you completed an incident report.

Telephone Communication

You will use the telephone to communicate with your supervisor. Always ask permission before using a client's phone. You may also need to answer the phone for your clients and know how to take messages.

When making a call, follow these steps:

1. Plan your call before you pick up the phone. This will help you be as efficient as possible.

2. Always identify yourself before asking to speak to someone. Never ask "Who is this?" when someone answers your call.

3. After you have identified yourself, ask for the person with whom you need to speak.

4. If the person you are calling is available, identify yourself again. State why you are calling.

5. If the person is not available, ask if you can leave a message. Always leave a message, even if it is only to say you called. The message shows that you were trying to reach someone.

6. Leave a brief and clear message. Do not give more information than necessary.

7. Thank the person who takes the message for you. Always be polite over the telephone, as you would in person.

Infection Prevention

This section provides a brief review of infection prevention, Standard Precautions, and Transmission-Based, or Isolation, Precautions. It is intended only as a brief review of concepts and skills with which you may already be familiar.

Preventing the spread of infection is as important in the home as in any other healthcare setting. The difference is that in the home, a great responsibility rests on the caregiver. There is no facility present to supply the proper equipment or enforce policies or procedures. Be familiar with the **infection control** practices of your agency. This includes all policies and procedures affecting your day-to-day tasks. There are no high faucets or deep sinks with special liquid soap and paper towel dispensers in most homes. You will be expected to adapt to what is actually available for your use. Therefore, assess the home for available infection control resources first. Plan how you will follow the appropriate standards of care. This includes the proper precautions to prevent and control infection.

Home Care Bag

In some situations, it may be a good idea for the HHA to carry a "home care bag." This bag can contain needed supplies, such as gloves, special handwashing wipes or soaps, paper towels, alcohol wipes, and a personal protective equipment (PPE) kit for emergencies. This special bag, such as a small duffel bag, should be used in place of a purse. A purse can become contaminated when carried from house to house. This bag should not be placed on the floor or on the client's bed or table. It should be placed on clean pieces of newspaper which the family can provide. Put it in an area close to where the client's care will be given. Designate this area as the "home care corner." This is an excellent spot to keep any other supplies caregivers might need as they care for the client. These include gloves, care plans, education materials, and dressings and tape.

Spread of Infection

Medical asepsis is the process of removing **pathogens**, or the state of being free of pathogens. It refers to the clean conditions you want to create in the home. Preventing the spread of infection is important. To understand how to prevent disease you must first know how it is spread. The chain of infection is a way of describing how disease is transmitted from one living being to another. Definitions and examples of the six links in the chain of infection are as follows:

Link 1: The **causative agent** is a pathogen or **microorganism** that causes disease. Causative agents include bacteria, viruses, fungi, and protozoa.

Link 2: A **reservoir** is where the pathogen lives and grows. Examples include the lungs, blood, and large intestine.

Link 3: The **portal of exit** is any body opening on an infected person that allows pathogens to leave, such as the nose, mouth, eyes, rectum, vagina, urethra, or a cut in the skin.

Link 4: The **mode of transmission** describes how the pathogen travels from one person to the next person. Transmission can happen through the air or by **direct contact** or **indirect contact**.

Link 5: The **portal of entry** is any body opening on an uninfected person that allows pathogens to enter. This can occur through the nose, mouth, eyes, other mucous membranes, a cut in the skin, or dry/cracked skin.

Link 6: A **susceptible host** is an uninfected person who could get sick. Examples include all healthcare workers and anyone in their care who is not already infected with that particular disease.

If one of the links in the chain of infection is broken, then the spread of infection is stopped.

Standard Precautions

The <u>Centers for Disease Control and Prevention</u> (CDC) is a federal government agency that issues information to protect the health of individuals and communities. In 1996, the CDC recommended a new infection control system to reduce the risk of contracting infectious diseases in healthcare settings. In 2007, some additions and changes were made to this system. There are two levels of precautions within the infection control system: Standard Precautions and Transmission-Based, or Isolation, Precautions.

Following **Standard Precautions** means treating all blood, body fluids, non-intact skin (like abrasions, pimples, or open sores), and **mucous membranes** (lining of mouth, nose, eyes, rectum, or genitals) as if they were infected. Standard Precautions are simple to remember because they include everything except sweat. Under Standard Precautions, "body fluids" include saliva, sputum (mucus coughed up), urine, feces, semen, vaginal secretions, and pus or other wound drainage.

Standard Precautions must be practiced on every single person in your care. This is the only safe way of doing your job. You cannot tell by looking at your clients or their medical charts if they have an **infectious** disease such as HIV, hepatitis, or influenza.

Standard Precautions include the measures below:

- **Wash your hands** before putting on gloves. Wash your hands immediately after removing gloves. Be careful not to touch clean objects with your used gloves.

- **Wear gloves** if you may come into contact with: blood; body fluids or secretions; broken skin, such as abrasions, acne, cuts, stitches or staples; or mucous membranes. Such contacts occur during mouth care; toilet assistance; perineal care; helping with a bedpan or urinal; ostomy care; cleaning up spills; cleaning basins, urinals, bedpans, and other containers that have held body fluids; and disposing of wastes.

- **Remove gloves** immediately when finished with a procedure.

- **Immediately wash all skin surfaces that have been contaminated** with blood and body fluids.

- **Wear a disposable gown** that is resistant to body fluids if you may come into contact with blood or body fluids.

- **Wear a mask and protective goggles** if you may come into contact with splashing or spraying blood or body fluids.
- **Wear gloves and use caution when handling razor blades, needles, and other sharps.** **Sharps** are needles or other sharp objects. Discard them carefully in a puncture-resistant biohazard container.
- **Never attempt to cap needles or sharps.** Dispose of them in a biohazardous waste container.
- **Avoid nicks and cuts** when shaving clients.
- **Carefully bag all contaminated supplies.** Dispose of them according to your agency's policy.
- **Clearly label body fluids** that are saved for a specimen with the client's name and a biohazard label. Keep them in a container with a lid.
- **Dispose of contaminated wastes** according to your agency's policy.

In your work you will use your hands constantly. Microorganisms are on everything you touch. Washing your hands is the single most important thing you can do to prevent the spread of disease. The CDC has defined **hand hygiene** as handwashing with either plain or antiseptic soap and water and using alcohol-based hand rubs.

Alcohol-based hand rubs include gels, rinses, and foams. They do not require the use of water. **Hand antisepsis** refers to washing hands with water and soap or other detergents that contain an antiseptic agent.

Alcohol-based hand rubs—often just called "hand rubs"—have proven effective in reducing bacteria on the skin. However, they are not a substitute for proper handwashing. Always use soap and water for visibly soiled hands. Once hands are clean, hand rubs can be used in addition to handwashing any time your hands are not visibly soiled. When using a hand rub, the hands must be rubbed together until the product has completely dried. Use hand lotion to prevent dry, cracked skin.

If you wear rings, consider removing them while working. Rings may increase the risk of contamination. Keep fingernails short, smooth, and clean. Do not wear artificial nails or extenders because they harbor bacteria and increase the risk of contamination. You should wash your hands:

- When arriving at a client's home
- Whenever they are visibly soiled
- Before and after all contact with a client
- Before and after making meals or working in the kitchen
- Before and after feeding a client

- After contact with any body fluids, mucous membranes, non-intact skin, or dressings
- After handling contaminated items
- Before putting on gloves and after removing gloves or any type of personal protective equipment (PPE)
- Before getting clean linen
- Before reaching into the clean area of your supply bag
- After touching garbage or trash
- After picking up anything from the floor
- Before and after you eat
- Before and after using the toilet
- After blowing your nose or coughing or sneezing into your hand
- After smoking
- After touching areas of your body, such as your mouth, face, eyes, hair, ears, or nose
- After any contact with pets and after contact with pet care items
- Before leaving a client's home

Washing hands

Equipment: soap, paper towels

1. Turn on water at sink. Keep your clothes dry, because moisture breeds bacteria.

2. Angle your arms down, holding your hands lower than your elbows. This prevents water from running up your arm. Wet hands and wrists thoroughly (Fig. 2-2).

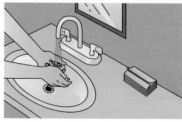

Fig. 2-2.

3. Apply a generous amount of soap to your hands.

4. Rub hands together and between each of your fingers to create a lather. Lather all surfaces of fingers and hands, including your wrists (Fig. 2-3). Use friction for at least 20 seconds. Friction helps clean.

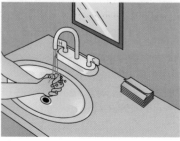

Fig. 2-3.

5. Clean your nails by rubbing them in the palm of your hand (Fig. 2-4).

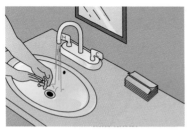

Fig. 2-4.

6. Being careful not to touch the sink, rinse thoroughly under running water. Rinse all surfaces of your hands and wrists. Run water down from wrists to fingertips. Do not run water over unwashed arms down to clean hands (Fig. 2-5).

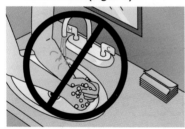

Fig. 2-5.

7. Use clean, dry paper towel to dry all surfaces of hands, wrists, and fingers. Do not wipe towel on unwashed forearms and then wipe clean hands. Dispose of towel without touching wastebasket. If your hands touch the sink or wastebasket, start over.

8. Use a clean, dry paper towel to turn off faucet (Fig. 2-6). Do not contaminate your hands by touching the surface of the sink or faucet.

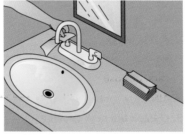

Fig. 2-6.

9. Dispose of used paper towel(s) in wastebasket after turning off faucet.

Personal Protective Equipment (PPE) 43

Personal protective equipment (PPE) is equipment that helps protect employees from serious injuries or illnesses resulting from contact with workplace hazards. Your employer is responsible for giving you the appropriate PPE to wear for client assignments.

44 Personal protective equipment includes gowns, masks, goggles, face shields, and gloves. Gowns protect the skin and/or clothing. Masks protect the mouth and nose. Goggles protect the eyes. Face shields protect the entire face—the mouth, nose, and eyes. Gloves protect the hands. Gloves are used most often by all caregivers.

You should wear PPE if there is a chance you could come into contact with body fluids, mucous membranes, or open wounds. Wear, or don, gowns, masks, goggles, and face shields when splashing or spraying of body fluids or blood could occur. When finished with a procedure, remove, or doff, the gown as soon as possible and wash your hands.

Putting on (donning) gown

1. Wash your hands.

2. Open gown. Hold out in front of you and allow gown to open/unfold (Fig. 2-7). Do not shake it. Slip your arms into the sleeves and pull the gown on.

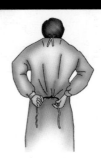

Fig. 2-8.

5. Use a gown only once and then remove and discard it. If gown becomes wet or soiled during care, remove it. Check clothing. Put on a new gown. The Occupational Safety and Health Administration (OSHA) requires non-permeable gowns—gowns that liquids cannot penetrate—when working in a bloody situation.

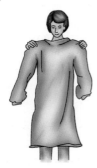

Fig. 2-7.

3. Fasten the neck opening.

4. Reach behind you. Pull gown until it completely covers your clothing. Secure gown at waist (Fig. 2-8).

6. Put on gloves after putting on gown.

When removing a gown, first remove gloves. Next, unfasten gown at neck and waist. Remove without touching outside of gown. Roll the dirty side in and away from the body.

42 Masks should be worn when caring for residents with respiratory illnesses. Always change masks when between clients; do not wear the same mask from one client to another. Goggles provide protection for your eyes.

Putting on (donning) mask and goggles

1. Wash your hands.

2. Pick up mask by top strings or elastic strap. Do not touch mask where it touches your face.

3. Adjust mask over your nose and mouth. Tie top strings

first, then bottom strings. Masks must always be dry or they must be replaced. Never wear a mask hanging from only the bottom ties (Fig. 2-9).

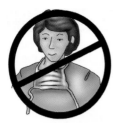

4. **Put on the goggles.**
5. **Put on gloves after putting on mask and goggles.**

Fig. 2-9.

When additional skin protection is needed, a face shield can be used as a substitute for wearing a mask or goggles. Follow your agency's policies.

Your agency will have specific policies and procedures on when to wear gloves. Learn and follow these rules. Always wear gloves for the following tasks:

- Any time you might touch blood or any body fluid, including vomitus, urine, feces, or saliva
- When performing or helping with mouth care or care of any mucous membrane
- When performing or helping with **perineal care** (care of the genital and anal area)
- When performing personal care on non-intact skin—skin that is broken by abrasions, cuts, rashes, acne, pimples, or boils
- When assisting with personal care when you have open sores or cuts on your hands
- When shaving a client
- When disposing of soiled bed linens, gowns, dressings, and pads

Clean, non-sterile gloves are generally adequate. They may be vinyl, latex, or nitrile; however, some people are allergic to latex. If you are, let your supervisor know. Your employer will provide you with gloves you can wear.

If you have cuts or sores on your hands, first cover these areas with bandages or gauze and then put on gloves. Disposable gloves are to be worn only once. They may not be washed or disinfected for reuse. Change gloves right before contact with mucous membranes or broken skin, or if gloves are soiled, torn, or damaged. Wash hands before putting on fresh gloves.

Putting on (donning) gloves

1. Wash your hands.

2. If you are right-handed, slide one glove on your left hand (reverse if left-handed).

3. With gloved hand, slide the other hand into the second glove.

4. Interlace fingers to smooth out folds and create a comfortable fit.

5. Carefully look for tears, holes, or spots. Replace the glove if necessary.

6. If wearing a gown, pull the cuff of the gloves over the sleeve of the gown (Fig. 2-10).

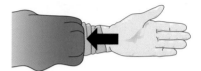

Fig. 2-10.

Remove gloves promptly after use. Remove your gloves before touching non-contaminated items or surfaces. Always wash your hands directly after removing gloves. You are wearing gloves to protect your skin from becoming contaminated. After giving care, your gloves are contaminated. If you open a door with the gloved hand, the doorknob becomes contaminated. Later, when you open the door with an ungloved hand, you will be infected. It is a common mistake to contaminate the room around you. Do not do it. Before touching surfaces, remove your gloves. Wash your hands. Afterward, put on new gloves if needed.

Removing (doffing) gloves

1. Touching only the outside of one glove, pull the first glove off by pulling down from the cuff (Fig. 2-11).

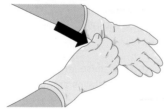

Fig. 2-11.

2. As the glove comes off your hand, it should be turned inside out.

3. With the fingertips of your gloved hand, hold the glove

you just removed. With your ungloved hand, reach two fingers *inside* the remaining glove, being careful not to touch any part of the outside of glove (Fig. 2-12).

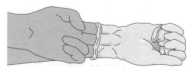

Fig. 2-12.

4. Pull down, turning this glove inside out and over the first glove as you remove it.

5. You should now be holding one glove from its clean inner side and the other glove should be inside it.

6. Drop both gloves into the proper container.

7. Wash your hands.

Special Precautions

Spills in the home, especially those involving blood, body fluids, or glass, can pose a serious risk of infection. Hospitals and long-term care settings have special types of flooring and specific commercial solutions they use for spills. In the home, such products may not be available. Read the labels of cleaning products carefully. Certain precautions may need to be taken with their use. For example, they may contain bleach that could take the color out of a carpet as well as removing the stain or spill.

Guidelines: Cleaning Spills Involving Blood, Body Fluids, or Glass

G   When blood or body fluids are spilled, put on gloves before starting to clean up the spill. In some cases, industrial-strength gloves are best.

G   If blood or body fluids are spilled on a hard surface such as a linoleum floor or countertop, clean immediately using a solution of one part household bleach to nine parts water. You can mix the solution in a bucket, and, with gloves on, wipe up the spill with rags or paper towels dipped in the solution. Be careful not to spill bleach or bleach solution on clothes, carpets, or bedding. It can discolor and damage fabrics. Your employer may provide commercial products for cleaning spills.

G   If blood or body fluids are spilled on fabrics such as carpets, bedding, or clothes, do not use bleach to clean the spill. Commercial disinfectants that do not contain bleach are available. If you have no disinfectant, wear gloves and wipe spills using soap and water. Then clean carpet with regular carpet cleaner. Use gloves to load soiled bedding or clothes into the washing machine and add color-safe bleach to the washer with the laundry detergent.

G   Do not pick up any pieces of broken glass, no matter how large, with your hands. Use a dustpan and broom or other tools.

G   Waste containing broken glass, blood, or body fluids should be properly bagged. Waste containing blood or body fluids may need to be placed in a special biohazard waste bag and disposed of separately from household trash. Follow your agency's policy.

Infectious Disease Precautions

Transmission-Based, or Isolation, Precautions are used when caring for persons who are infected or suspected of being infected with a disease. When ordered, these precautions are used in addition to Standard Precautions. These precautions will always be listed in the care plan and on your assignment sheet. It is for your safety and the safety of others that these precautions must be followed.

Guidelines: Infectious Diseases

G Always follow Standard Precautions.

G Wash your hands frequently, especially after client care.

G Use gloves, gowns, masks, and goggles when needed.

G Follow isolation procedures described in the assignment sheet for each client.

G Handle laundry, personal items, and waste carefully.

There are three categories of Transmission-Based Precautions. The category used depends on the disease and how it spreads. They may also be used in combination for diseases that have multiple routes of transmission. Transmission-Based Precautions are always used **in addition** to Standard Precautions.

Airborne Precautions

Airborne Precautions are used for diseases that can be transmitted through the air after being expelled. The pathogens are so small that they can attach to moisture in the air. They remain floating for some time. For certain care you will be required to wear a N95 mask or a HEPA respirator to avoid infection. Airborne diseases include tuberculosis, measles, and chickenpox.

Droplet Precautions

Droplet Precautions are used when the disease-causing microorganism does not remain in the air. These pathogens usually travel only short distances after being expelled. Droplets normally do not travel more than three feet. Droplets can be created by coughing, sneezing, talking, laughing, or suctioning. Droplet Precautions include wearing a face mask during care and restricting visits from uninfected people. Cover your nose and mouth with a tissue when you sneeze or cough. Ask clients, family, and others to do the same. Dispose of the tissue in the nearest waste container. If you sneeze on your hands, wash them promptly. An example of a droplet disease is the mumps.

Contact Precautions

Contact Precautions are used when there is a risk of transmitting or contracting a microorganism from touching an infected object or person. Lice, scabies (a skin disease that causes itching), and bacterial conjunctivitis (pink eye) are examples of situations that require Contact Precautions. Transmission can occur with skin-to-skin contact during transfers or bathing. Contact Precautions include wearing PPE and client isolation. They require washing hands with **antimicrobial** soap. They also require not touching infected surfaces with ungloved hands or uninfected surfaces with contaminated gloves.

Two important points to remember are:

1 When they are indicated, Transmission-Based Precautions are always used **in addition** to Standard Precautions.

2 The client must be reassured that it is the disease, not the person with the disease, that is being isolated. Talk with your client. Explain why these special steps are being taken.

MRSA

MRSA stands for methicillin-resistant *Staphylococcus aureus*. *Staphylococcus aureus* is a common type of bacteria that can cause illness. Methicillin is a powerful antibiotic drug. MRSA is an antibiotic-resistant infection often acquired in hospitals and other facilities. MRSA infections also occur in otherwise healthy people who have not been recently hospitalized. They are sometimes acquired in fitness centers when equipment has not been disinfected during use. These infections are known as community-associated MRSA infections (CA-MRSA) and are usually skin infections, such as pimples or boils.

MRSA can spread among those having close contact with infected people. It is almost always spread by direct physical contact, and not through the air. If a person has MRSA on his skin, especially on the hands, and touches someone, he may spread MRSA. Spread also occurs through indirect contact by touching objects, such as sheets or clothes, contaminated by the infected skin of a person with MRSA.

To help prevent MRSA practice good hygiene. Handwashing, using soap and warm water, is the single most important measure to control MRSA. Keep cuts and abrasions clean and covered with a proper dressing (e.g. bandage) until healed. Avoid contact with other people's wounds or material that is contaminated from wounds.

Several state and federal government agencies have guidelines and laws concerning infection control. **OSHA** requires employers to provide for the safety of their employees through rules and suggested guidelines. The Centers for Disease Control issues guidelines for healthcare workers to follow on the job. Some of the infection control requirements for you and your employer are listed below.

Employer's responsibilities for infection control include the following:

- Establish infection control procedures and an **exposure control plan** to protect workers.

- Provide continuing in-service education on infection control, including education on airborne and **bloodborne pathogens** and updates on any new safety standards.

- Provide PPE for employees to use and train them on when and how to properly use it.

- Provide free hepatitis B vaccinations for all "at-risk employees." As a home health aide, you are considered at-risk.

Employee's responsibilities for infection control include the following:

- Follow Standard Precautions.

- Follow all agency policies and procedures.

- Follow client care plans and assignments.

- Use provided PPE as indicated or appropriate.

- Take advantage of the free hepatitis B vaccination.

- Immediately report any exposure you have to infection, blood, or body fluids.

- Participate in annual education programs covering infection control.

Safety and Body Mechanics

Principles of Body Mechanics

Back strain or injury is one of the greatest risks that home health aides face. Using proper body mechanics is an important step in preventing back strain and injury. **Body mechanics** is the way the parts of the body work together whenever you move. Understanding some basic principles of body mechanics will help keep you and clients safe.

Alignment. When standing, sitting, or lying down, try to have your body in alignment. This means that the two sides of the body are mirror images of each other, with body parts lined up naturally. Maintain correct body alignment when lifting or carrying an object by keeping the object close to your body. Point your feet and body in the direction you are moving. Avoid twisting at the waist.

Base of support. The base of support is the foundation that supports an object. The feet are the body's base of support. The wider your support, the more stable you are. Standing with your legs shoulder-width apart allows for a greater base of support. You will be more stable than someone standing with his feet together.

Center of gravity. The center of gravity in your body is the point where the most weight is concentrated. This point will depend on the position of the body. When you stand, your weight is centered in your pelvis. A low center of gravity gives a more stable base of support. Bending your knees when lifting an object lowers your pelvis and, therefore, lowers your center of gravity. This gives you more stability and makes you less likely to fall or strain the working muscles.

Some examples of using proper body mechanics include the following:

When lifting a heavy object from the floor, spread your feet shoulder-width apart and bend your knees. Using the strong, large muscles in your thighs, upper arms, and shoulders, lift the object. Pull it close to your body, level with your pelvis. By doing this, you keep the object close to your center of gravity and base of support. When you stand up, push with your strong hip and thigh muscles. Raise your body and the object together.

Do not twist when you are moving an object. Always face the object or person you are moving. Pivot your feet instead of twisting at the waist.

To help a client sit up, stand up, or walk, protect yourself by assuming a good stance. Place your feet about 12 inches or shoulder-width, apart. Put one foot in front of the other, with your knees bent. Your upper body should stay upright and in alignment. Do this whenever you have to support a client's weight. If the client starts to fall, you will be in a good position to help support him or her. Never try to catch a falling client. If a client falls, assist him or her to the floor. If you try to reverse a fall in progress, you will probably injure yourself and/or the client.

Bend your knees to lower yourself, rather than bending from the waist. When a task requires bending, use a good stance. This lets you use the big muscles in your legs and hips rather than the smaller muscles in your back.

If you are making an adjustable bed, adjust the height to a safe working level, usually waist high. Avoid bending at the waist.

Keep the following tips in mind to avoid strain and injury:

- Assess the situation first. Clear the path. Remove any obstacles.
- Use both arms and hands to lift, push, or carry objects.
- Hold objects close to you when you are lifting or carrying them.
- Push objects and equipment rather than lifting them.
- Avoid bending and reaching as much as possible. Move or position furniture so that you do not have to bend or reach.
- Avoid twisting at the waist. Instead, turn your whole body. Your feet should point toward what you are lifting.
- When moving a client, let him know what you will do so he can help if possible. Count to three. Lift or move on three so everyone moves together.
- Report to your supervisor if your assignments include tasks you feel you cannot safely perform. Never attempt to lift an object or a client that you feel you cannot handle.

Following are several strategies that can help you apply good body mechanics in the home:

- **Have the right tools for a job**. For example, if you cannot reach an object on a high shelf, use a step stool rather than climbing on a counter or straining to reach.
- **Have footrests and pillows available**. For example, tasks that require standing for long periods can be more comfortable if you rest one foot on a footrest. This position flexes the muscles in the lower back and keeps the spine in alignment. When sitting, using a footrest allows for a more comfortable leg position. Crossing the legs disrupts alignment. It should be avoided. Using pillows can make any chair more comfortable. Use pillows behind the back to keep the back straight.
- **Keep tools, supplies, and clutter off the floor**. Keep frequently-used items on shelves or counters where they can be easily reached without lifting. Keeping things organized will also help you find what you need without straining.
- **Sit when you can**. Whenever you can sit to do a job, do so. Chopping vegetables, folding clothes, and other tasks can be done easily while sitting. For jobs like scouring the bathtub, kneel or use a low stool. Avoid bending at the waist.

- **Use gait or transfer belts when assisting clients with ambulation or transfers.** In Section IV, you will learn correct procedures for safely assisting clients with ambulation and transfers.

Accident Prevention

Falls: Falls are among the most common home accidents. Falls can be caused by an unsafe environment or by loss of abilities. Falls are particularly common among the elderly. Older people are often more seriously injured by falls because their bones are more fragile. Be especially alert to the risk of falls with your elderly clients.

Factors that raise the risk of falls include:
- Clutter
- Throw rugs
- Exposed electrical cords
- Slippery floors
- Uneven floors or stairs
- Poor lighting

Personal conditions that raise the risk of falls include medications, loss of vision, gait or balance disturbances, weakness, paralysis, and disorientation. **Disorientation** means confusion about person, place, or time.

Follow these guidelines to guard against falls:

- Clear all walkways of clutter, throw rugs, and cords.
- Avoid waxing floors, and use non-skid mats or carpeting where appropriate.
- Have clients wear non-skid shoes. Make sure shoelaces are tied.
- Have clients wear clothing that fits properly, e.g. is not too long.
- Keep frequently-used personal items close to the client.
- Immediately clean up spills on the floor.
- Mark uneven flooring or stairs with red tape to indicate a hazard.
- Improve lighting where necessary.

Burns/Scalds: Burns can be caused by dry heat (hot iron, stove, other electrical appliances), wet heat (hot water or other liquids, steam), or chemicals (lye, acids). Small children, older adults, or people with loss of sensation due to paralysis are at greatest risk of burns. Scalds are burns caused by hot liquids. It takes five seconds or less for a serious burn to occur when the temperature of liquid is 140°F. Coffee, tea, and other hot drinks are usually served at 160°F to 180°F. Follow these guidelines to guard against burns and scalds:

- Roll up sleeves and avoid loose clothing when working at the stove.
- Check that the stove and appliances are off when you leave.
- Suggest that the hot water heater be set lower than normal. It should be set at 120°F to 130°F to avoid burns from scalding tap water.
- Always check water temperature with water thermometer or on your wrist before using.
- Check temperatures of liquids on your wrist before serving.
- Keep space heaters away from clients' beds, chairs, and draperies. Never allow space heaters to be used in the bathroom.
- Report frayed electrical cords or unsafe-looking appliances immediately. Do not use these appliances.
- Let clients know you are about to pour or set down a hot liquid.
- Pour hot drinks away from clients. Keep hot drinks and liquids away from edges of tables. Put a lid on them.
- Make sure clients are sitting down before serving hot drinks.

Poisoning: Homes contain many harmful substances that should not be swallowed. These include cleaning products, paints, medicines, toiletries, and glues. Follow these guidelines to guard against poisoning:

- Lock harmful products away from confused clients, clients with limited vision, and children.
- Have the number for the Poison Control Center posted by the telephone.
- Check the refrigerator and cabinets frequently for foods that are moldy, sour, or spoiled. Investigate any odors you notice.

Cuts: Cuts typically occur in the kitchen or bathroom. Follow these guidelines to guard against cuts:

- Keep any sharp objects, including knives, peelers, graters, food processor blades, scissors, nail clippers, and razors out of reach of children.
- Lock sharp objects away if there is a confused client in the home.
- If you are preparing food, cut away from yourself, use a cutting board, and keep your fingers out of the way.
- Know proper first aid for cuts.

444

44444

Choking: Choking can occur when eating, drinking or swallowing medication. Babies and young children who put objects in their mouths are at great risk of choking. People who are weak, ill, or unconscious may choke on their own saliva. A person's tongue can also become swollen and obstruct the airway. Follow these guidelines to guard against choking:

- Keep small objects out of reach of babies and small children.
- Cut food into bite-sized pieces for clients who have trouble with utensils and for children.
- Position infants on their backs for sleeping after feeding. Infants should sleep on their backs to prevent sudden infant death syndrome (SIDS). Never put pillows, small toys, or other objects in a crib.
- Clients should eat in as upright a position as possible to avoid choking. Elderly clients with swallowing difficulties may have a special diet with liquids thickened to the consistency of honey or syrup. Thickened liquids are easier to swallow. See Section VI for more information on swallowing problems and thickened liquids.

Fire: Follow these guidelines to guard against fire:

- Roll up clients' sleeves and avoid loose clothing when clients may be cooking or around the stove.
- Store potholders, dish towels, and other flammable kitchen items away from the stove.
- Never store cookies, candy, or other items that may attract children above or near the stove.
- Discourage careless smoking and smoking in bed. If clients must smoke, check to be sure that cigarettes are extinguished. Empty ashtrays frequently. Before emptying ashtrays, make sure there are no hot ashes or hot matches in ashtray.
- Stay in or near the kitchen when anything is cooking or baking.
- Do not leave the dryer on when you leave the house. Lint can catch fire.
- Turn off space heaters when no one is home or everyone is asleep.
- Be sure there are working smoke alarms.
- Have fire extinguishers on hand. Every home should have a fire extinguisher in the kitchen. Check that the homes you work in have fire extinguishers that have not expired. Know where fire extinguisher is stored and how to operate it. The PASS acronym will help you understand how to use it:

- **P**ull the pin.
- **A**im at the base of the fire when spraying.
- **S**queeze the handle.
- **S**weep back and forth at the base of the fire.
- In case of fire, the RACE acronym is a good rule to follow:
  - **R**emove clients from danger.
  - **A**ctivate 911.
  - **C**ontain fire if possible.
  - **E**xtinguish, or call fire department to extinguish.

In addition, follow these guidelines for helping clients and family members exit the home safely:

- Remain calm.
- Be sure all family members know how to exit in case of fire, and have a designated meeting place outside the home.
- If windows or doors have locking bars, keep keys in the lock or close by. Mark windows of children's rooms with stickers that indicate a child sleeps in the room.
- Remove anything blocking a window or door that could be used as a fire exit.
- Stay low in a room to escape a fire.
- Use a covering over the face to reduce smoke inhalation.
- If clothing catches fire, do not run. Stop, drop to the ground, and roll to extinguish flames.
- If door is closed, check for heat coming from it before opening it. If the door or doorknob feels hot to the touch, it is best to stay in the room if there is no safe exit. Plug the doorway (use wet towels or clothing) to prevent smoke from entering. Stay in the room until help arrives.

Travel Safety

Since you may be driving to and from clients' homes, you will need to protect your safety. Follow these guidelines:

- **Plan your route**. Trying to read a map or directions while driving can be very dangerous. When you must drive to a new location, study the map or directions before you start your car.

- **Minimize distractions**. Paying attention to the road can help you avoid accidents. Keep your eyes on the road and your hands on the wheel. If music is distracting, do not listen in the car. Do not talk on your cell phone. Do not send text messages or read incoming text messages.
- **Use turn signals**. Using your turn signals lets other drivers know what you are planning to do. Always use turn signals when preparing to turn or change lanes.
- **Use caution when backing up**. Many accidents occur when drivers back up. When you back up, look around you carefully. Turn your head to both sides and look behind your car.
- **Drive at a safe speed**. Follow speed limits to be sure you are not driving too fast. Road conditions such as ice or heavy rain may mean you have to drive at a slower speed.
- **Always wear your seat belt**. Although it may not help you avoid an accident, it will certainly help protect you if an accident occurs.
- **Keep your driver's license, valid car insurance, and proof of registration with you** in case you're ever in an accident or stopped by police.

If an assignment takes you to an area where crime is a problem, use caution. If you are using public transportation, be alert at all times. Follow these guidelines to help avoid trouble:

- Park in well-lit areas as close as possible to the home you are visiting.
- Try to leave valuables at home when you must work in a dangerous area.
- If possible, do not take your purse with you. If you must take it, hold your purse or bag tightly, close to your body.
- Lock your car and do not leave any valuables in it.
- Walk confidently. Look as though you know where you are going.
- Carry a whistle so you can make a loud noise to startle an attacker and get help.
- Carry your keys in your hand to unlock your car as soon as you arrive.
- Do not sit in your car, even with the doors locked. Drive away as soon as you reach your car.
- Try to avoid unsafe areas after dark.
- If you are concerned about your safety in a particular area, leave the area immediately. Contact your supervisor.
- Do not approach a home where strangers are hanging around. Go to your car and drive to a safe area. Use your cell phone or the nearest phone in a safe area, and call your supervisor.

- Call your client before you visit so he or she knows approximately when to expect you.
- Never enter a vacant home.
- If necessary, ask your supervisor to arrange for an escort or another care provider to go with you.
- Be sure someone knows your schedule. Call the office at the end of your work day.

Emergencies

Medical Emergencies

Medical emergencies may be caused by accidents or sudden illnesses. This section discusses what to do in a medical emergency. Heart attacks, stroke, diabetic emergencies, choking, automobile accidents, and gunshot wounds are all medical emergencies. Falls, burns, and cuts can also be emergencies.

In an emergency, try to remain calm, act quickly, and communicate clearly. Knowing these steps will help:

Assess the situation. Try to find out what has happened. Make sure you are not in danger. Notice the time.

Assess the victim. Ask the injured or ill person what has happened. If the person cannot respond, he may be unconscious. Determine whether or not the person is conscious. Tap the person and ask if he is all right. Speak loudly. Use the person's name if you know it. If there is no response, assume the person is unconscious. This is an emergency. Call for help right away, or send someone else to call.

If a person is conscious and able to speak, then he is breathing and has a pulse. Talk with the person about what happened. Get the person's permission to touch him or her. Check the person for injury. Look for severe bleeding, changes in consciousness, irregular breathing, unusual color or feel to the skin, swollen places on the body, medical alert tags, and anything the client says is painful. If any of these exist, you may need medical help. Always get help before doing anything else.

If the injured or ill person is conscious, he may be frightened. Listen to the person. Tell him what is being done to help him. Be calm and confident. Reassure him that you are taking care of him.

When in doubt about calling for help, call! If you need to call emergency medical services, dial 911. If you are alone, make the call yourself. If you are not alone, shout for help and have someone make the call for you and then return to assist you.

When calling emergency services, be prepared to give the following information:

- The phone number and address of emergency, including exact directions or landmarks if necessary
- The person's condition, including any medical background you know
- Your name and position
- Details of any first aid being given

The dispatcher you speak with may need other information or may want to give you other instructions. Do not hang up the phone until the dispatcher hangs up or tells you to hang up. If you are in a home, unlock the front door so emergency personnel can get in when they arrive.

If the person is breathing, has a normal pulse, is normally responsive, and is not bleeding severely, you may not need to call for emergency services. If a client has fallen, been burned, or cut himself but the damage seems to be minor, call your supervisor. Let the person answering the phone know that you are with a client and that an accident has occurred. If your supervisor is not available, another member of the care team may be able to help you.

Once the emergency is over, you will need to document it in your notes. Complete an incident report. Try to remember as many details as possible. Only report the facts, not opinions. Knowing what information you will have to document will help you remember the important facts. Documenting emergencies accurately is very important to you and your agency.

First aid is emergency care given immediately to an injured person. **Cardiopulmonary resuscitation** (**CPR**) is the medical procedures used when a person's heart or lungs have stopped working. CPR is used until medical help arrives. Quick action is necessary. CPR must be started immediately. Only properly trained people should perform CPR. Your agency will probably arrange for you to be trained in CPR. If not, ask about American Heart Association or Red Cross CPR training, or contact one of these agencies yourself. CPR is an important skill to learn. If you are not trained, do not attempt to perform CPR. Performing CPR incorrectly can further injure a person.

Choking

When something is blocking the tube through which air enters the lungs, the person has an obstructed airway. When people are choking, they usually put their hands to their throats (Fig 2-13). As long as a person can speak, breathe, or cough, do nothing. Encourage her to cough as forcefully as possible to get the object out. Stay with the person at all times, until she stops choking or can no longer speak, breathe, or cough. Do not hit her on the back. If a person can no longer speak, breathe, or cough, or turns blue,

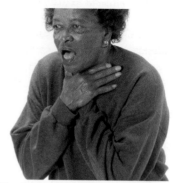

Fig. 2-13. *People who are choking usually put their hands to their throats.*

call 911 immediately. After calling 911, return to the person. Time is of extreme importance.

Abdominal thrusts are a method of attempting to remove an object from the airway of someone who is choking. These thrusts work to remove the blockage upward, out of the throat. Make sure the person needs help before starting to give abdominal thrusts. Ask, "Can you cough? Can you speak? Can you breathe? Are you choking?" Say, "I know what to do. Can I help you?" This is obtaining consent. If the person cannot speak or cough, or if his response is weak, start giving abdominal thrusts.

Performing abdominal thrusts for the conscious person

1. Stand behind the person. Bring your arms under her arms. Wrap your arms around the person's waist.

2. Make a fist with one hand. Place the flat, thumb side of the fist against the person's abdomen, above the navel but below the breastbone.

3. Grasp the fist with your other hand. Pull both hands toward you and up, quickly and forcefully.

4. Repeat until the object is pushed out or the person loses consciousness.

5. Report and document the incident properly.

Insulin Reaction and Diabetic Ketoacidosis

Insulin reaction (also called hypoglycemia) can result from either too much insulin or too little food. It occurs when insulin is given, and the person skips a meal or does not eat all the food required. Even when a regular amount of food is eaten, physical activity may rapidly absorb the food. This causes too much insulin to be in the body. Vomiting and diarrhea may also lead to insulin shock in people with diabetes.

The first signs of insulin reaction include feeling weak or different, nervousness, dizziness, and perspiration (see list below for further signs). These signal that the client needs food in a form that can be rapidly absorbed. A lump of sugar, a hard candy, or a glass of orange juice should be consumed right away. A diabetic should always have a quick source of sugar handy. Contact your supervisor if the client has shown early signs of insulin reaction. Other signs and symptoms of insulin reaction include:

- Hunger
- Weakness
- Rapid pulse
- Headache
- Low blood pressure
- Cold, clammy skin
- Confusion
- Trembling
- Nervousness
- Blurred vision
- Numbness of the lips and tongue
- Unconsciousness

Diabetic ketoacidosis (DKA) (also called hyperglycemia) is caused by having too little insulin. It can result from undiagnosed diabetes, going without insulin or not taking enough, eating too much, not getting enough exercise, or physical or emotional stress. The signs of the onset of diabetic ketoacidosis include increased thirst or urination, abdominal pain, deep or labored breathing, and breath that smells sweet or fruity (see list below for further signs). Call your supervisor immediately if you suspect your client is experiencing diabetic ketoacidosis. Other signs and symptoms of diabetic ketoacidosis include the following:

- Hunger
- Weakness
- Rapid, weak pulse
- Headache
- Low blood pressure

- Dry skin
- Flushed cheeks
- Drowsiness
- Nausea and vomiting
- Air hunger, or client gasping for air and being unable to catch his breath
- Unconsciousness

Refer to the Special Conditions section for more information on diabetes.

CVA or Stroke

A **cerebrovascular accident** (**CVA**), or stroke, is caused when blood supply to the brain is suddenly cut off by a clot or a ruptured blood vessel. A quick response to a suspected stroke is critical. Tests and treatment need to be given within a short time of the stroke's onset. Early treatment may be able to reduce the severity of the stroke.

A transient ischemic attack, or TIA, is a warning sign of a CVA. It is the result of a temporary lack of oxygen in the brain. Symptoms may last up to 24 hours. They include difficulty speaking, weakness on one side of the body, temporary loss of vision, and numbness or tingling. These symptoms should not be ignored. Report any of these to your supervisor immediately. These are also signs that a CVA is occurring:

- Facial numbness or weakness, especially on one side
- Arm numbness or weakness, especially on one side
- Slurred speech or difficulty speaking
- Use of inappropriate words
- Inability to understand spoken or written words
- Redness in the face
- Noisy breathing
- Dizziness
- Blurred vision
- Ringing in the ears
- Headache
- Nausea/vomiting
- Seizures

- Loss of bowel and bladder control
- Paralysis on one side of the body
- Elevated blood pressure
- Slow pulse rate
- Loss of consciousness

Refer to the Special Conditions section for more information on strokes.

Myocardial Infarction or Heart Attack

Myocardial infarction (**MI**), or heart attack, occurs when the heart muscle itself does not receive enough oxygen because blood vessels are blocked. A myocardial infarction is an emergency that can result in serious heart damage or death. The following are signs and symptoms of MI:

- Sudden, severe pain in the chest, usually on the left side or in the center, behind the breastbone
- Pain or discomfort in other areas of the body, such as one or both arms, the back, neck, jaw, or stomach
- Indigestion or heartburn
- Nausea and vomiting
- **Dyspnea**, or difficulty breathing
- Dizziness
- Pale, gray, or **cyanotic** (bluish) skin, indicating lack of oxygen
- Perspiration
- Cold and clammy skin
- Weak and irregular pulse rate
- Low blood pressure
- Anxiety and a sense of doom
- Denial of a heart problem

The pain of a heart attack is commonly described as a crushing, pressing, squeezing, stabbing, piercing pain, or, "like someone is sitting on my chest." The pain may go down the inside of the left arm. A person may also feel it in the neck and/or in the jaw. The pain usually does not go away.

As with men, women's most common symptom is chest pain or discomfort. But women are somewhat more likely than men to have shortness of breath, nausea/vomiting, and back, shoulder, or jaw pain. Some women's symptoms seem more flu-like, and women are more likely to deny that they are having a heart attack.

You must take immediate action if a resident has any of these symptoms. Follow these steps:

Responding to a heart attack

1. **Call or have someone call emergency services. Call your supervisor.**

2. **Place the person in a comfortable position. Encourage him to rest, and reassure him that you will not leave him alone.**

3. **Loosen clothing around the neck.**

4. **Do not give the person liquids or food.**

5. **If the person takes heart medication, such as nitroglycerin,** find the medication and offer it to him. Never place medication in someone's mouth.

6. **Monitor the person's breathing and pulse. If the person stops breathing or has no pulse, perform CPR only if you are trained to do so.**

7. **Stay with the person until help arrives.**

8. **Report and document the incident properly.**

Refer to the Special Conditions section for more information on heart attacks.

Disaster Guidelines

Disasters can include fire, flood, earthquake, hurricane, tornado, or severe weather. Acts of terrorism may also be considered disasters. The disasters you may experience will depend on where you live. Know the appropriate action to take to protect yourself and your client. During natural disasters, most agencies rely on local or state management groups and the American Red Cross to assume overall responsibility for the ill and disabled. Each agency has a local and area-specific disaster plan readily available for employees to learn. Know your agency's disaster plan. The following guidelines apply in any disaster situation:

• Remain calm.

• Listen to radio or television bulletins to keep informed. A battery-powered radio will help you to stay informed if power goes out.

• If a disaster is forecast (for example, a tornado or hurricane), be ready. Wear appropriate clothing and shoes. Have family members dressed and ready in case evacuation is necessary.

• Stay in contact with your supervisor or others if possible. Let someone know where you are, what conditions exist, and where you will go if you must evacuate.

- Locate disaster supplies. Ideally, a disaster supplies kit should be assembled before disaster strikes. See below.

Emergency Supplies

Keep enough supplies in your home to meet your needs for at least three days. Assemble a disaster supply kit with items you may need in an evacuation. Store kit in sturdy, easy-to-carry containers such as backpacks, duffel bags, or covered trash containers.

Include:

- A three-day supply of water (one gallon per person per day) and food that will not spoil
- One change of clothing and footwear per person, and one blanket or sleeping bag per person
- A first aid kit that includes your family's prescription medications
- Emergency tools, including a battery-powered radio, flashlight, and plenty of extra batteries
- An extra set of car keys and a credit card, cash, or traveler's checks
- Sanitation supplies
- Special items for infant, elderly, or disabled family members
- An extra pair of glasses
- Important family documents in a waterproof container

You will be required to apply general guidelines as well as specific guidelines for the area in which you work. For example, a HHA working where hurricanes occur, such as Florida, needs to know the guidelines for hurricanes preparedness, as well as for storms and fires. The following guidelines are separated by the type of disaster. They can be used in any particular geographical area that applies to your specific job and location. Always keep the radio or television on to get the latest information.

Tornadoes

In the case of tornadoes, follow these guidelines:

- Seek shelter inside, such as steel-framed or concrete buildings.
- Stay away from windows.
- Go to the hallway or basement, or take cover under heavy furniture.
- Do not stay in a mobile home or trailer.
- Lie as flat as possible.

Lightning

If outdoors, follow these guidelines:

- Avoid the largest objects, such as trees and open spaces.
- Stay out of the water.
- Seek shelter in buildings.
- Stay away from metal fences, doors, or other objects.
- Avoid holding metal objects in your hands, such as golf clubs.
- Stay in automobiles.
- CPR is safe to perform because lightning victims carry no electricity.

If indoors, stay inside and away from open doors and windows. Avoid using electrical equipment such as hair dryers and televisions. Do not use the phone.

Floods

In the case of floods, follow these guidelines:

- Fill the bathtub with fresh water.
- Board up windows.
- Evacuate if advised to do so.
- Check the fuel level in automobiles.
- Have a portable battery-operated radio, flashlight, and cooking equipment available.
- Do not drink water or eat food that has been contaminated with flood water.
- Do not handle electrical equipment.
- Do not turn off gas yourself, but ask the gas company to do so.

Blackouts

In the case of blackouts, follow these guidelines:

- In a facility you will have access to either a generator or a flashlight.
- In a home, ask your client where the emergency supplies are kept. Take prompt action to keep calm and provide light.
- Use a back-up pack for electrical medical equipment such as an IV pump. Back-up packs do not last more than 24 hours, so call emergency services.

Hurricanes

In the case of hurricanes, follow these guidelines:

- Know what category the hurricane is and track the expected path.
- Know which clients must go to shelters, nursing homes, or hospitals, and which need special assistance.
- Call your employer for instructions.
- Contact your clients if instructed to do so.
- Fill the bathtub with fresh water.
- Board up windows.
- Evacuate if advised to do so.
- Check the fuel level in automobiles.
- Have a portable battery-operated radio, flashlight, and cooking equipment available.
- Be aware of people with special needs.
- High-risk people include the elderly and those unable to evacuate on their own. High-risk areas include mobile homes or trailers.

III.
Understanding Your Clients

Culture and Family

Basic Human Needs

People have different genes, physical appearances, cultural backgrounds, ages, and social or financial positions. But all human beings have the same basic physical needs:

- Food and water
- Protection and shelter
- Activity
- Sleep and rest
- Safety
- Comfort, especially freedom from pain

People also have **psychosocial needs**, which involve social interaction, emotions, intellect, and spirituality. Psychosocial needs are not as easy to define as physical needs. However, all human beings have the following psychosocial needs:

- Love and affection
- Acceptance by others
- Security
- Self-reliance and independence in daily living
- Contact with other people
- Success and self-esteem

Health and well-being affect how well psychosocial needs are met. Stress and frustration occur when basic needs are not met. This can lead to fear, anxiety, anger, aggression, withdrawal, indifference, and depression. Stress can also cause physical problems that may eventually lead to illness.

Abraham Maslow, a researcher of human behavior, wrote about human physical and psychosocial needs. He arranged these needs into an order of importance. He thought that physical needs must be met before psychosocial needs can be met. His theory is called "Maslow's Hierarchy of Needs" (Fig. 3-1)

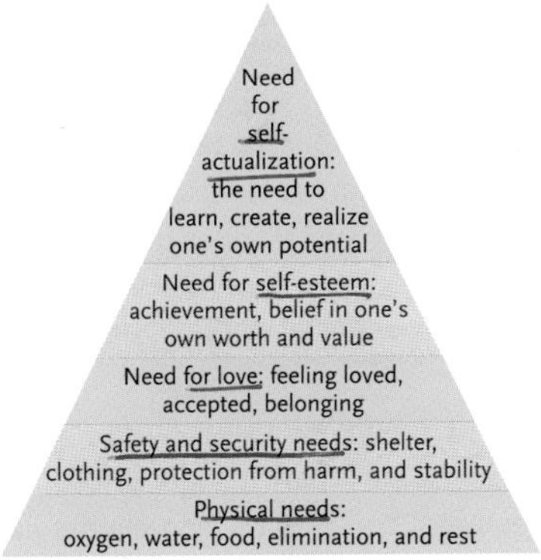

Need for self-actualization: the need to learn, create, realize one's own potential

Need for self-esteem: achievement, belief in one's own worth and value

Need for love; feeling loved, accepted, belonging

Safety and security needs: shelter, clothing, protection from harm, and stability

Physical needs: oxygen, water, food, elimination, and rest

Fig. 3-1. *Maslow's Hierarchy of Needs.*

Cultural Differences

People come from many different cultural backgrounds and traditions. You will take care of clients with different backgrounds and traditions than your own. It is important to respect and value each person as an individual. Sometimes it is easier to accept different practices or beliefs if you understand a little about them.

There are so many different cultures that they cannot all be listed here. A **culture** is a system of learned behaviors, practiced by a group of people, that are considered to be the tradition of that people and are passed on from one generation to the next. Each culture may have different knowledge, behaviors, beliefs, values, attitudes, religions, and customs. One might talk about American culture being different from Japanese culture. But within American culture there are thousands of different groups with their own cultures. Japanese-Americans, African-Americans, and Native Americans are just a few. Even people from a particular region, state, or city can be said to have a different culture. The culture of the South is not the same as the culture of New York City.

Cultural background affects how friendly people are to strangers. It can affect how they feel about having you in their houses, or how close they want you to stand to them when talking. It can affect how they feel about you performing care for them or discussing their health with them. Be sensitive to your clients' backgrounds and preferences. You cannot expect to be treated the same way by all your clients. You may have to adjust your behavior around some clients. Treat all clients with respect and professionalism. Expect them to treat you respectfully as well.

Religious differences also influence the way people behave. Religion can be very important in people's lives, particularly when they are ill or dying. You must respect the religious beliefs and practices of your clients, even if they are different from your own. Never question your clients' religious beliefs. Do not discuss your own beliefs with them.

Be aware of specific practices that affect your work. Many religious beliefs include dietary restrictions. These are rules about what and when followers can eat and drink. Check with your agency if you are unsure about planning and preparing meals for clients. Be aware of any dietary restrictions. Honor them.

Some people's backgrounds may make them less comfortable being touched. Ask permission before touching clients. Be sensitive to their feelings. You must touch clients in order to do your job. However, recognize that some clients feel more comfortable when there is little physical contact.

Families

Families are the most important unit within our social system. Families play a huge role in most people's lives. Some examples of family types are listed below:

- Single-parent families include one parent with a child or children.
- Nuclear families include two parents with a child or children.
- Blended families include widowed or divorced parents who have remarried. There may be children from previous marriages as well as from this marriage.
- Multigenerational families include parents, children, and grandparents.
- Extended families may include aunts, uncles, cousins, or even friends.
- Families may also be made up of unmarried couples of the same sex or opposite sexes, with or without children.

Family members help in many ways:

- Helping clients make care decisions
- Communicating with the care team
- Providing daily care when home health aide is not present
- Giving support and encouragement
- Connecting the client to the outside world
- Giving assurance to dying clients that family memories and traditions will be valued and carried on

Body Systems

Each system in the body has a condition under which it works best. **Homeostasis** is the name for the condition in which all of the body's systems are working their best. To be in homeostasis, the body's **metabolism**, or physical and chemical processes, must be working at a steady level. When disease or injury occur, the body's metabolism is disturbed. Homeostasis is lost. Changes in metabolic processes are called signs and symptoms. Each system in the body has its own unique structure and function. Body systems can be broken down in different ways. In this book we divide the human body into ten body systems:

1. Integumentary, or skin

2. Musculoskeletal

3. Nervous

4. Circulatory or Cardiovascular

5. Respiratory

6. Urinary

7. Gastrointestinal

8. Endocrine

9. Reproductive

10. Immune and Lymphatic

Body systems are made up of organs. An organ has a specific function. Organs are made up of tissues. Tissues are made up of groups of cells that perform a similar task. For example, in the circulatory system, the heart is one of the organs. It is made up of tissues and cells. Cells are the building blocks of bodies. Living cells divide, develop, and die, renewing the tissues and organs of the body.

Common Disorders/Observing and Reporting

1. The Integumentary System

The largest organ and system in the body is the skin. Skin is a natural protective covering, or integument. It prevents injury to internal organs. It also protects the body against entry of bacteria or germs. Skin also prevents the loss of too much water, which is essential to life. Skin is made up of layers of tissue. Within these layers are sweat glands, which secrete sweat to help cool the body when needed, and sebaceous glands, which secrete oil (sebum) to keep the skin lubricated. There are also hair follicles, many tiny blood vessels (capillaries), and tiny nerve endings.

The skin is also a sense organ. It feels heat, cold, pain, touch, and pressure. It then tells the brain what it is feeling. Body temperature is regulated in the skin. Blood vessels **dilate** when the outside temperature is too high. This brings more blood to the body surface to cool it off. The same blood vessels **constrict** when the outside temperature is too cold. By restricting the amount of blood reaching the skin, the blood vessels help the body retain heat.

Common Disorders: Integumentary System

C/D Pressure sores, or decubitus ulcers

Observing and Reporting : Integumentary System

During daily care, a client's skin should be observed for changes that may indicate injury or disease. Observe and report these signs and symptoms:

O/R Pale, white, reddened, or purple areas

O/R Blisters or bruises

O/R Dry or flaking skin

O/R Rashes or any skin discoloration

O/R Cuts, boils, sores, wounds, abrasions

O/R Fluid or blood draining from the skin

O/R Changes in moistness/dryness

O/R Swelling

O/R Changes in wound or ulcer (size, depth, drainage, color, odor)

O/R Redness or broken skin between toes or around toenails

O/R Scalp or hair changes

O/R Skin that appears different from normal or that has changed

O/R In ebony complexions, also look for any change in the feel of the tissue, any change in the appearance of the skin, such as an "orange-peel" look, a purplish hue, and extremely dry, crust-like areas that might be covering a tissue break.

2. The Musculoskeletal System

Muscles, bones, ligaments, tendons, and cartilage give the body shape and structure. They work together to move the body. Exercise is important for improving and maintaining both physical and mental health. Range of motion (ROM) exercises can help prevent loss of self-esteem, depression, pneumonia, urinary tract infection, constipation, blood clots, dulling of the senses, and muscle **atrophy** or **contractures**.

Common Disorders: Musculoskeletal System

C/D **Fractures**

C/D **Osteoporosis**

C/D Arthritis

Observing and Reporting: Musculoskeletal System

Observe and report the following signs and symptoms:

O/R Changes in ability to perform routine movements and activities

O/R Any changes in clients' ability to perform ROM exercises

O/R Pain during movement

O/R Any new or increased swelling of joints

O/R White, shiny, red, or warm areas over a joint

O/R Bruising

O/R Aches and pains reported to you

3. The Nervous System

The nervous system is the control center and message center of the body. It controls and coordinates all body functions. The nervous system also senses and interprets information from the environment outside the human body.

Common Disorders: Central Nervous System

C/D **Dementia**, including Alzheimer's disease

C/D Cerebrovascular accident (CVA), or stroke

C/D Parkinson's disease

C/D **Multiple sclerosis**

C/D **Epilepsy**

C/D Cerebral palsy

C/D Head and spinal cord injuries

Observing and Reporting: Central Nervous System

Observe and report the following signs and symptoms:

O/R Fatigue or pain with movement or exercise

O/R Shaking or trembling

O/R Inability to speak clearly

O/R   Inability to move one side of body

O/R   Disturbance or change in vision or hearing

O/R   Changes in eating patterns or fluid intake

O/R   Difficulty swallowing

O/R   Bowel and bladder changes

O/R   Depression or mood changes

O/R   Memory loss or confusion

O/R   Violent behavior

O/R   Any unusual or unexplained change in behavior

O/R   Decreased ability to perform ADLs

The Nervous System: Sense Organs

The eyes, ears, nose, tongue, and skin are the body's major sense organs. They are part of the central nervous system because they receive impulses from the environment. They relay these impulses to the nerves.

Common Disorders: Eyes and Ears

C/D   Cataracts

C/D   **Glaucoma**

C/D   Otitis media (infection of the middle ear)

C/D   Deafness

C/D   Vertigo (dizziness)

Observing and Reporting: Eyes and Ears

Observe and report the following signs and symptoms:

O/R   Changes in vision or hearing

O/R   Signs of infection

O/R   Dizziness

O/R   Complaints of pain in eyes or ears

4. The Circulatory or Cardiovascular System

The circulatory system is made up of the heart, blood vessels, and blood. The heart pumps blood through the blood vessels to the cells. The blood carries food, oxygen, and other substances that cells need to function properly.

The circulatory system supplies food, oxygen, and hormones to cells. It supplies the body with infection-fighting blood cells. It removes waste products from cells. The circulatory system also controls body temperature.

Common Disorders: Circulatory System

- C/D Atherosclerosis (hardening and narrowing of the blood vessels)
- C/D Myocardial infarction (MI), or heart attack
- C/D Angina pectoris (chest pain, pressure, or discomfort)
- C/D Hypertension, or high blood pressure
- C/D Congestive heart failure (heart is no longer able to pump effectively)
- C/D Peripheral vascular disease (poor circulation to extremities)

Observing and Reporting: Circulatory System

Observe and report the following signs and symptoms:

- O/R Changes in pulse rate
- O/R Weakness, fatigue
- O/R Loss of ability to perform activities of daily living (ADLs)
- O/R Swelling of hands and feet
- O/R Pale or bluish hands, feet, or lips
- O/R Chest pain
- O/R Weight gain
- O/R Shortness of breath, changes in breathing patterns, or inability to catch breath
- O/R Severe headache
- O/R Inactivity (which can lead to circulatory problems)

5. The Respiratory System

Respiration, the body taking in oxygen and removing carbon dioxide, involves breathing in (inspiration), and breathing out (expiration). The lungs accomplish this process. The functions of the respiratory system are to bring oxygen into the body and to eliminate carbon dioxide produced as the body uses oxygen.

Common Disorders: Respiratory System

- C/D **Asthma**
- C/D Upper respiratory infection (URI), or a cold

C/D **Chronic obstructive pulmonary disease (COPD)**

C/D **Bronchitis**

C/D Pneumonia

C/D Emphysema

C/D Lung cancer

C/D **Tuberculosis**

Observing and Reporting: Respiratory System

Observe and report the following signs and symptoms:

O/R Change in respiratory rate

O/R Shallow breathing or breathing through pursed lips

O/R Coughing or wheezing

O/R Nasal congestion or discharge

O/R Sore throat, difficulty swallowing, or swollen tonsils

O/R The need to sit after mild exertion

O/R Pale or bluish color of the lips and arms and legs

O/R Pain in the chest area

O/R Discolored **sputum** (green, yellow, blood-tinged, or gray)

6. The Urinary System

The urinary system is composed of two kidneys, two ureters, one urinary bladder, and a single urethra. The urinary system has two important functions. Through urine, the urinary system eliminates waste products created by the cells. The urinary system also maintains the water balance in the body.

Common Disorders: Urinary System

C/D Urinary incontinence

C/D Urinary tract infection (UTI), or cystitis

C/D Calculi (kidney stones)

C/D Nephritis (inflammation of the kidneys)

C/D Renovascular hypertension

C/D Chronic kidney failure, or chronic renal failure

Observing and Reporting: Urinary System

Observe and report the following signs and symptoms:

O/R   Weight loss or gain

O/R   Swelling in the upper or lower extremities

O/R   Pain or burning during urination

O/R   Changes in urine, such as cloudiness, odor, or color

O/R   Changes in frequency and amount of urination

O/R   Swelling in the abdominal/bladder area

O/R   Complaints that bladder feels full or painful

O/R   Urinary incontinence/dribbling

O/R   Pain in the kidney or back/flank region

O/R   Inadequate fluid intake

7. The Gastrointestinal (GI) System

The gastrointestinal (GI) system, also called the digestive system, is made up of the gastrointestinal tract and the accessory digestive organs. The gastrointestinal system has two functions: **digestion** and **elimination**.

Common Disorders: Gastrointestinal System

C/D   Heartburn

C/D   **Gastroesophageal reflux disease (GERD)**

C/D   Peptic ulcers

C/D   **Constipation**

C/D   **Diarrhea**

C/D   **Hepatitis**

C/D   Ulcerative colitis

C/D   Colitis

C/D   Colorectal cancer

C/D   Hemorrhoids

Observing and Reporting: Gastrointestinal System

Observe and report the following signs and symptoms:

O/R   Difficulty swallowing or chewing (including denture problems, tooth pain, or mouth sores)

○/R   Fecal incontinence (inability to control the bowels, leading to involuntary passage of stool)

○/R   Weight gain/weight loss

○/R   Anorexia (loss of appetite)

○/R   Abdominal pain and cramping

○/R   Diarrhea

○/R   Nausea and vomiting (especially vomitus that looks like coffee grounds)

○/R   Constipation

○/R   Flatulence/gas

○/R   Hiccups or belching

○/R   Bloody, black, or hard stools

○/R   Heartburn

○/R   Poor nutritional intake

8. The Endocrine System

The endocrine system is made up of glands that secrete hormones. **Glands** are structures in the body that produce substances. Each substance has a specific purpose in the overall functioning of the body. **Hormones** are chemical substances created by the body that regulate essential body processes. They are carried in the blood to the organs, where they perform these functions:

• Maintaining homeostasis

• Influencing growth and development

• Regulating levels of sugar in the blood

• Regulating levels of calcium in the bones

• Regulating the body's ability to reproduce

• Determining how fast cells burn food for energy

Common Disorders: Endocrine System

C/D   Hyperthyroidism

C/D   Hypothyroidism

C/D   Diabetes

Observing and Reporting: Endocrine System

Observe and report the following signs and symptoms:

O/R   Blurred vision*

O/R   Dizziness*

O/R   Sweating/excessive perspiration*

O/R   Change in "normal" behavior*

O/R   Confusion*

O/R   Change in mobility*

O/R   Change in sensation*

O/R   Numbness or tingling in arms or legs*

O/R   Headache

O/R   Weakness

O/R   Hunger

O/R   Irritability

O/R   Weight gain/weight loss

O/R   Loss of appetite/increased appetite

O/R   Increased thirst

O/R   Frequent urination or any change in urine output

O/R   Dry skin

O/R   Skin breakdown

O/R   Sweet or fruity breath

O/R   Sluggishness or fatigue

O/R   Hyperactivity

* indicates signs and symptoms that should be reported immediately

9. The Reproductive System

The reproductive system is made up of the reproductive organs, which are different in men and women. The reproductive system allows human beings to reproduce, or create new human life. Reproduction begins when a male's and female's sex cells (sperm and ovum) join. These sex cells are formed in the male and female sex glands, called the gonads.

Common Disorders: Reproductive System

C/D   Vaginitis

C/D   Benign prostatic hypertrophy

C/D Chlamydia

C/D Syphilis

C/D Gonorrhea

C/D Herpes simplex 2

Observing and Reporting: Reproductive System

Observe and report the following signs and symptoms:

O/R Discomfort or difficulty with urination

O/R Discharge from the penis or vagina

O/R Swelling of the genitals

O/R Blood in urine or stool

O/R Breast changes (in both males and females), including size, shape, lumps, or discharge from the nipple

O/R Sores on the genitals

O/R Client reports of impotence, or inability of male to have sexual intercourse

O/R Client reports of painful intercourse

10. *The Immune and Lymphatic Systems*

The immune system protects the body from disease-causing bacteria, viruses, and organisms in two ways. Nonspecific immunity protects the body from disease in general. Specific immunity protects against a particular disease that is invading the body at a given time.

The lymphatic system removes excess fluids and waste products from the body's tissues. It also helps the immune system fight infection.

Common Disorders: Immune and Lymphatic Systems

C/D **HIV/AIDS**

C/D Lymphoma

Observing and Reporting: Immune and Lymphatic Systems

Observe and report the following signs and symptoms immediately:

O/R Recurring infections (such as diarrhea and fevers)

O/R Swelling of the lymph nodes

O/R Increased fatigue

Human Development

Stages/Common Disorders

Everyone will go through the same stages of development during their lives. However, no two people will follow the exact same pattern or rate of development. Each client must be treated as an individual and as a whole person who is growing and developing, rather than someone who is merely ill or disabled.

Infancy, Birth to 12 Months

Infants grow and develop very quickly. In one year a baby moves from total dependence on the caregiver to the relative independence of moving around, communicating basic needs, and feeding himself.

Physical development in infancy moves from the head down. For example, infants gain control over the muscles of the neck before they are able to control the muscles in their shoulders. Control over muscles in the trunk area, such as the shoulders, develops before control of the arms and legs. This head-to-toe sequence should be respected when caring for infants. For example, newborns must be supported at the shoulders, head, and neck. Babies who cannot sit or crawl should not be encouraged to stand or walk.

Common Disorders: Infancy

- ℅ Prematurity
- ℅ Low birth weight
- ℅ Birth defects: cerebral palsy, cystic fibrosis, Down syndrome
- ℅ Viral or bacterial infections
- ℅ Sudden infant death syndrome (SIDS)

Childhood

The Toddler Period, Ages 1 to 3

During the toddler years, children gain independence. One part of this independence is new control over their bodies. Toddlers learn to speak, gain coordination of their limbs, and gain control over their bladders and bowels. Toddlers assert their new independence by exploring. Poisons and other hazards, such as sharp objects, must be locked away.

Psychologically, toddlers learn that they are individuals, separate from their parents. Children of this age may try to control their parents. They may try to get what they want by throwing tantrums, whining, or refusing to cooperate. This is a key time for parents to set rules and standards.

The Preschool Years, Ages 3 to 6

Children in their preschool years develop skills that will help them become more independent and have social relationships. They develop vocabulary and language skills. They learn to play in groups. They become more physically coordinated, and learn to care for themselves. Preschoolers also develop ways of relating to family members. They begin to learn right from wrong.

School-Age Children, Ages 6 to 12

From ages 6 to about 12 years, children's development is centered on **cognitive** (related to thinking and learning skills) and social development. As children enter school, they also explore the environment around them. They relate to other children through games, peer groups, and classroom activities. In these years, children learn to get along with each other. They also begin to behave in ways common to their gender. They begin to develop a conscience, morals, and self-esteem.

Common Disorders: Childhood

C/D Chickenpox

C/D Viral or bacterial infections

C/D Leukemia

C/D Child abuse

Adolescence

Puberty

During puberty, secondary sex characteristics, such as body hair, appear. Reproductive organs begin to function. The body begins to secrete reproductive hormones. The start of puberty occurs between the ages of 10 and 16 for girls and 12 and 14 for boys.

Adolescence, Ages 12 to 18

Many teenagers have a hard time adapting to the changes that occur in their bodies during puberty. Peer acceptance is important to them. Adolescents may be afraid that they are ugly or even abnormal. This concern for body image and acceptance, combined with changing hormones that influence emotions, can cause rapid mood swings. Adolescents need to express themselves socially and sexually. This can cause conflict and stress. Social interaction between members of the opposite sex becomes very important.

Common Disorders: Adolescence

ᶜ/ᴅ Eating disorders: **anorexia**, bulimia

ᶜ/ᴅ **Sexually transmitted infections (STIs)** and **sexually transmitted diseases (STDs)**

ᶜ/ᴅ Teenage pregnancy

ᶜ/ᴅ Depression

ᶜ/ᴅ Trauma or accidental injury

Adulthood

Young Adulthood, Ages 18 to 40

By the age of 18, most young adults have stopped growing. Adopting a healthy lifestyle in these years can make life better now and prevent health problems in later adulthood. Psychological and social development continues, however. The tasks of these years include choosing an appropriate education and an occupation or career, selecting a mate, learning to live with a mate or others, raising children, and developing a satisfying sex life.

Middle Adulthood, Ages 40 to 65

In general, people in middle adulthood are more comfortable and stable than they were before. Many of their major life decisions have already been made. In the early years of middle adulthood people sometimes experience a "mid-life crisis." This is a period of unrest centered around a subconscious desire for change and for fulfillment of unmet goals.

Late Adulthood, Ages 65 Years and Older

Persons in late adulthood must adjust to the effects of aging. These effects or changes can include the loss of strength and health, death of loved ones, retirement, and preparation for death. The developmental tasks of this age seem to deal entirely with loss. But solutions to these problems often involve new relationships, friendships, and interests.

The disorders you are most likely to see in this age group are discussed in Section V.

Aging

Aging causes many changes. However, normal changes of aging do not mean an older person must become dependent, ill, or inactive. Knowing how to tell normal changes of aging from signs of illness or disability will allow you to better help clients. Normal changes of aging include:

- Skin is thinner, drier, more fragile, and less elastic.
- Muscles weaken and lose tone.
- Bones become more brittle.
- Sensitivity of nerve endings in the skin decreases.
- Responses and reflexes slow.
- Short-term memory loss occurs.
- Senses of vision, hearing, taste, and smell weaken.
- Heart works less efficiently.
- Oxygen in the blood decreases.
- Appetite decreases.
- Urinary elimination is more frequent.
- Digestion takes longer and is less efficient.
- Levels of hormones decrease.
- Immunity weakens.
- Lifestyle changes occur.

There are also changes which are NOT considered normal changes of aging and should be reported to your supervisor. These include:

- Signs of depression
- Suicidal thoughts
- Loss of ability to think logically
- Disorientation
- Confusion
- Poor nutrition
- Shortness of breath
- Incontinence

Keep in mind that this is not a complete list. Your job includes reporting any change, normal or not.

Death

Death can occur suddenly and without warning, or it can be expected. Older people, or people with terminal illnesses, may have time to prepare for death. A **terminal illness** is a disease or condition that will eventually cause death. Preparing for death is a process that involves the dying person's emotions and behavior.

Dr. Elisabeth Kubler-Ross researched and wrote about the process of dying. Her book, *On Death and Dying*, describes five stages that dying people and their families or friends may experience before death. These five stages are described below.

- **Denial**: People in the denial stage may refuse to believe they are dying. They often believe a mistake has been made.

- **Anger**: Once they start to face the possibility of their death, people may become angry that they are dying.

- **Bargaining**: Once people have begun to believe that they are dying, they may make promises to God. They may somehow try to bargain for their recovery.

- **Depression**: As dying people become weaker and symptoms get worse, they may become deeply sad or depressed.

- **Acceptance**: Many people who are dying are eventually able to accept death and prepare for it. They may make plans for their last days or for the ceremonies to follow.

Death is a very sensitive topic. Many people find it hard to discuss. Feelings and attitudes about death can be formed by many factors:

- Experience with death
- Personality type
- Religious beliefs
- Cultural background

Common signs of approaching death include the following:

- Blurred and failing vision
- Unfocused eyes
- Impaired speech
- Diminished sense of touch
- Loss of movement, muscle tone, and feeling
- A rising or below-normal body temperature
- Decreasing blood pressure
- Weak pulse that is abnormally slow or rapid
- Slow, irregular respirations or rapid, shallow respirations
- Cold, pale skin
- Mottling (bruised appearance), spotting, or blotching of skin caused by poor circulation

- Perspiration
- Incontinence
- Disorientation or confusion

Guidelines: Caring for the Dying Client

G **Diminished senses**: Reduce glare and keep room lighting low. Hearing is usually the last sense to leave the body. Speak in a normal tone. Tell person about any procedures that are being done. Describe what is happening in the room. Do not expect an answer. Observe body language to anticipate client's needs.

G **Care of the mouth and nose**: Give mouth care often. If client is unconscious, give mouth care every two hours. Apply lubricant, such as lip balm, to the lips and nose.

G **Skin care**: Give bed baths and incontinence care as needed. Bathe perspiring clients often. Skin should be kept clean and dry. Change sheets and clothes for comfort. Keep sheets wrinkle-free. Reposition clients often. Skin care to prevent pressure sores is important.

G **Comfort**: Pain relief is critical. Observe for signs of pain and report them. Frequent changes of position, back massage, skin care, mouth care, and proper body alignment may help.

G **Environment**: Display favorite objects and photographs for client. Make sure room is appropriately lighted and well-ventilated.

G **Emotional and spiritual support**: Listen to client if she wishes to talk. Touch is important. Do not avoid the dying person or his or her family. Do not deny that death is approaching. Do not tell the client that anyone knows how or when it will happen. Some clients may seek spiritual comfort from clergy members. Give privacy for visits from clergy, family, and friends. Do not discuss your religious or spiritual beliefs with clients or their families or make recommendations.

Guidelines: Postmortem Care

G Bathe the body. Be gentle to avoid bruising. Place drainage pads where needed. Follow Standard Precautions.

G Check with family about how to dress client and whether or not to remove jewelry.

G Do not remove any tubes or other equipment.

G Put dentures back in the mouth and close the mouth.

G Close the eyes carefully.

G Position the body on the back with legs straight and arms folded across the abdomen. Place a small pillow under the head.

G Strip the bed after body has been removed.

G Open windows to air room, as appropriate, and straighten up.

G Arrange personal items carefully so they are not lost.

G Document according to your agency's policy.

Respect the wishes of family and friends. Be sensitive to their needs after death occurs. Only perform assigned tasks.

Dealing with grief after the death of a loved one is an individual process. No two people will grieve in exactly the same way. Clergy, counselors, or social workers can provide help for people who are grieving. Family members or friends may have any of these reactions to the death of a loved one:

- Shock
- Denial
- Anger
- Guilt
- Regret
- Sadness
- Loneliness

Hospice Care

Hospice is the term for the special care that a dying person needs. It is a compassionate way to care for dying people and their families. Hospice care uses a holistic approach. It treats the person's physical, emotional, spiritual, and social needs. Hospice care can be given seven days a week, 24 hours a day. Hospice care may be given in a hospital, at a care facility, or in the home. A hospice can be any location where a person who is dying is treated with dignity by caregivers.

Hospice care helps to meet all needs of the dying person. Family and friends, as well as the client, are directly involved in care decisions. The client is encouraged to participate in family life and decision-making as long as possible.

Home care differs from hospice care. In home care, goals will focus on the client's recovery, or on the client's ability to care for him- or herself as much as possible. In hospice care, however, the goals of care are the comfort and dignity of the client. This is an important difference. This type of care is called **palliative care**. You will need to adjust your mindset when caring for hospice clients. Focus on relieving their pain and making them comfortable, rather than on teaching them to care for themselves.

Clients who are dying also need to feel some independence for as long as possible. Caregivers should allow clients to retain as much control over their lives as possible. Eventually, caregivers may have to meet all of the client's basic needs.

Family members or friends who are caregivers for the dying person will appreciate your help. You are providing them with a break. This kind of care is sometimes referred to as respite care. You must be aware of the feelings of family caregivers. Encourage them to take breaks and take care of themselves. However, do not insist that they do so. Many want to do all they can for their loved one during his or her last days. Do observe family caregivers for signs of excessive stress. Report any signs to your supervisor. Your agency may be able to refer them to local support services.

Certain attitudes and skills are useful in hospice care:

- Be a good listener. Do not push someone to talk, though.
- Respect privacy and independence.
- Be sensitive to individual needs. Ask how you can be of help.
- Be aware of your own feelings.
- Follow the plan of care.
- Take good care of yourself.
- Allow yourself to grieve.

IV.
Client Care

Maintaining Mobility, Skin, and Comfort

Positioning

Clients who spend a lot of time in bed often need help getting into comfortable positions. They also need to change positions periodically to avoid muscle stiffness and skin breakdown or pressure sores. Bed-bound clients should be repositioned every two hours. Document the time and position with each change.

Following are the five basic body positions:

1. Supine, or lying flat on back (Fig. 4-1)

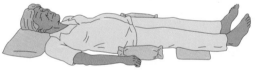

Fig. 4-1. *A person in the supine position is lying flat on his or her back.*

2. Lateral, or side (Fig. 4-2)

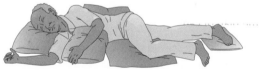

Fig. 4-2. *A person in the lateral position is lying on his or her side.*

3. Prone, or lying on the stomach (Fig. 4-3)

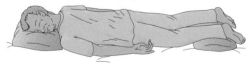

Fig. 4-3. *A person in the prone position is lying on his or her stomach.*

4. Fowler's, or semi-sitting position (45 to 60 degrees) (Fig. 4-4)

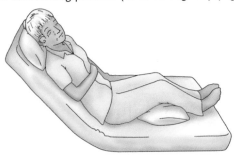

Fig. 4-4. *A person lying in the Fowler's position is partially reclined.*

5. Sims', or lying on the left side with one leg drawn up (Fig. 4-5)

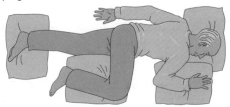

Fig. 4-5. *A person lying in the Sims' position is lying on his or her left side with one leg drawn up.*

Clients who are confined to bed need to maintain proper body alignment. This promotes recovery and prevents injury to muscles and joints. These guidelines help clients maintain good alignment and make progress when they can get out of bed:

Guidelines: Alignment and Positioning

G Observe principles of alignment. Proper alignment is based on straight lines. The spine should be in a straight line. Pillows or rolled or folded blankets can support the small of the back and raise the knees or head in the supine position. They can support the head and one leg in the lateral position.

G Keep body parts in natural positions. In a natural hand position, the fingers are slightly curled. Use a rolled washcloth, gauze bandage, or a rubber ball inside the palm to support the fingers in this position. Use bed cradles to keep covers from resting on feet in the supine position. Use footboards to keep the client's feet properly aligned.

G Prevent external rotation of hips. When legs and hips are allowed to turn outward during prolonged bed rest, hip contractures can result. A rolled blanket or towel that is tucked alongside the hip and thigh can keep the leg from turning outward.

G Change positions often to prevent muscle stiffness and pressure sores. This should be done at least every two hours. The position used depends on the client's condition and preference. Check the skin every time you reposition a client.

G Have plenty of pillows available to provide support in the various positions.

G Use positioning devices (backrests, bed cradles, **draw sheets**, footboards, and handrolls).

G Splints may be prescribed by a doctor to keep a client's joints in the correct position.

G Give back rubs for comfort and relaxation.

For more information on using positioning devices for comfort, refer to the Comfort Measures section.

Always use good body mechanics when moving or positioning a client. Avoid lifting whenever possible. Instead, push, roll, slide, or pivot, so that you are not bearing the client's weight. Using good body mechanics helps protect both you and your clients.

Helping a client sit up using the arm lock

1. Wash your hands.

2. Explain the procedure to the client, speaking clearly, slowly, and directly. Maintain face-to-face contact whenever possible.

3. Provide privacy if the client desires it.

4. If the bed is adjustable, adjust bed to a safe working level, usually waist high. If the bed is movable, lock bed wheels.

5. Stand facing the head of the bed, with your legs about 12 inches apart and your knees bent (Fig. 4-6).

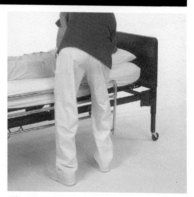

Fig. 4-6. Keeping your legs apart and knees bent helps prevent injury.

6. Place your arm under the client's armpit and grasp the client's shoulder. Have the client grasp your shoulder in the same manner. This hold is called the arm lock or lock arm (Fig. 4-7).

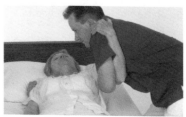

Fig. 4-7. Grasp the client's shoulder and have the client grasp yours.

7. Reach under the client's head and place your other hand on the client's far shoulder. Bend your knees.

8. At the count of three, rock yourself backward and pull the client to a sitting position. Use pillows or a bed rest to support the client in the sitting position.

9. Check the client for dizziness or weakness.

10. If you raised an adjustable bed, return it to its lowest position.

11. Wash your hands.

12. Document the procedure and any observations. Was the client able to help at all? Did the client become dizzy?

Before a client who has been lying down moves to a standing position, she should dangle. To **dangle** means to sit up with the feet over the side of the bed for a moment to regain balance. It gives the client time to adjust to being in an upright position after lying down. For some clients who are unable to walk, sitting up and dangling the legs for a few minutes may be ordered.

Assisting a client to sit up on side of bed: dangling

Equipment: non-skid footwear

1. Wash your hands.

2. Explain the procedure to the client, speaking clearly, slowly, and directly. Maintain face-to-face contact whenever possible.

3. Provide privacy if the client desires it.

4. If the bed is adjustable, adjust bed to lowest position. If the bed is movable, lock bed wheels.

5. Fanfold (fold into pleats) the top covers to the foot of the bed.

6. Raise the head of the bed to a sitting position.

7. Stand with your legs about 12 inches apart, with one foot 6-8 inches in front of the other. Bend your knees.

8. Place one arm under the client's shoulder blades. Place the other arm under the client's thighs (Fig. 4-8).

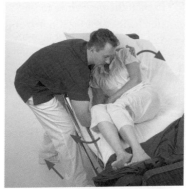

Fig. 4-8. Place one hand under the shoulder blades and the other under the thighs.

9. On the count of three, slowly turn client into a sitting position with legs dangling over the side of the bed. (Fig. 4-9).

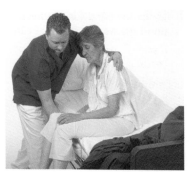

Fig. 4-9. *The weight of the client's legs hanging down from the bed helps the client sit up.*

10. Ask client to hold on to edge of mattress with both hands. Put non-skid shoes on the client while she is dangling. Do not leave the client alone. If the client is dizzy for more than a minute, have her lie down again. Take her pulse and respirations and report to your supervisor according to your agency's policy.

11. The care plan may direct you to allow the client to dangle for several minutes and then return her to lying down, or it may direct you to allow the client to dangle in preparation for walking or a transfer. Follow the instructions in the care plan.

12. Wash your hands after the transfer is completed.

13. Document the procedure and your observations. How did the client tolerate sitting up? Did the client become dizzy?

Transfers/Ambulation

Transferring a client means that you are moving him or her from one place to another. Transfers can move a client from a wheelchair to a bed, from a bed to a chair, and so on. Safety is one of the most important things to consider during transfers.

A **transfer belt** is a safety device used to transfer clients who are weak, unsteady, or uncoordinated. It is called a **gait belt** when used to help clients walk. The belt is made of canvas or other heavy material. It sometimes has handles and fits around the client's waist outside the clothing. The transfer belt is a safety device that gives you something firm to hold on to. When applying a transfer belt, place the belt over the client's clothing and around the waist. Do not put it over bare skin. Tighten the buckle until it is snug. Leave enough room to insert two fingers comfortably into the belt. For female clients, make sure the breasts are not caught under the belt.

Guidelines: Wheelchairs

G   Learn how a wheelchair works. Know how to apply and release the brake and how to operate the armrests and footrests. Lock the wheelchair before assisting a client into or out of it. After the transfer, unlock the wheelchair.

G   To transfer to or from a wheelchair, use the stronger side of the client's body that can bear weight to support the weaker side that cannot bear weight.

G   Before any transfer, make sure the client is wearing non-skid footwear which is securely fastened. This promotes the client's safety and reduces the risk of falls.

G   Make sure the client is safe and comfortable during transfers. Ask the client how you can help. Some clients may only want you to bring the chair to the bedside. Others may want you to be more involved.

G   When a client is in a wheelchair or any chair, he or she should be repositioned every two hours or as needed.

G   Keep the client's body in good alignment while in a wheelchair or chair. Special cushions and pillows can be used for support. The hips should be positioned well back in the chair. If the client needs to be moved back in the wheelchair, go to the back of the chair. Gently reach forward and down under the client's arms. Ask the client to place his feet on the ground and push up. Gently pull the client up in the chair while the client pushes.

Falls

Remember the following if a client starts to fall during a transfer:

- Widen your stance. Bring the client's body close to you to break the fall. Bend your knees and support the client as you lower her to the floor. You may need to drop to the floor with the client to avoid injury to you or the client.

- Do not try to reverse or stop a fall. You or the client can be injured if you try to stop rather than break the fall.

- Call for help if a family member is around. Do not try to get the client up after the fall unless you are certain the client is not injured. Many agencies do not allow helping a client up after a fall until she has been evaluated by a nurse. Follow your agency's policies and procedures. Always call your supervisor if you are unsure of what to do.

- If you do help the client up, get her in bed, take her vital signs, then report the fall to your supervisor immediately.

Transferring a client from bed to wheelchair or chair

Equipment: wheelchair, transfer belt, non-skid footwear

1. Wash your hands.

2. Explain the procedure to the client, speaking clearly, slowly, and directly. Maintain face-to-face contact whenever possible.

3. Provide privacy if the client desires it. Check the area to be certain it is uncluttered and safe.

4. Remove both wheelchair footrests close to the bed.

5. Place wheelchair or chair near the head of the bed with arm of the wheelchair almost touching the bed. The wheelchair or chair should be placed on client's stronger, or unaffected, side.

6. If using a wheelchair, lock the wheels.

7. If bed is adjustable, raise the head of the bed. Adjust the bed level so that the height of the bed is equal to or slightly higher than the chair. If bed is movable, lock bed wheels.

8. Assist client to sitting position with feet flat on the floor.

9. Put non-skid footwear on client and securely fasten.

10. *With transfer (gait) belt:*

    a. Stand in front of client.

    b. Stand with feet about 12 inches apart. Bend your knees.

    c. Place belt around client's waist over clothing (not on bare skin). Grasp belt securely on both sides.

Without transfer belt:

    a. Stand in front of client.

    b. Stand with feet about 12 inches apart. Bend your knees.

    c. Place your arms around client's torso under the arms. Ask client to use the bed to push up (or your shoulders, if possible).

11. Provide instructions to allow client to help with transfer. Instructions may include:

    "When you start to stand, push with your hands against the bed."

    "Once standing, if you're able, you can take small steps in the direction of the chair."

    "Once standing, reach for the chair with your stronger hand."

12. With your legs, brace client's lower legs to prevent slipping. This can be done by placing both of your knees in front of the client's knees. It can also be done by placing both of your knees on the outside of both of the client's legs. Follow agency policy.

13. Count to three to alert client. On three, slowly help client to stand.

14. Tell the client to take small steps in the direction of the chair while turning her back toward the chair. If more help is needed, help the client to pivot to front of wheelchair or chair with back of her legs against chair (Fig. 4-10).

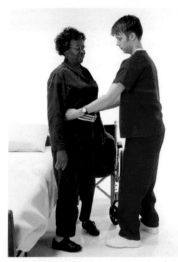

Fig. 4-10. Help her pivot to the front of the wheelchair, so that the back of her legs are against wheelchair.

15. Ask the client to put hands on wheelchair or chair arm rests if able. When the chair is touching the back of the client's legs, help her lower herself into the chair.

16. Reposition client with hips touching back of wheelchair or chair. Remove transfer belt, if used.

17. If using wheelchair, attach footrests. Place the client's feet on the footrests. Check that the client is in good alignment.

18. Wash your hands.

19. Document the procedure and your observations. How did the client feel or appear during the transfer? How much assistance was required?

A slide, or transfer, board may be used to help transfer clients who are unable to bear weight on their legs. Slide boards can be used for almost any transfer that involves moving from one sitting or reclining position to another. For example, slide boards can be helpful for transfers from bed to chair, wheelchair to bathtub, or wheelchair to car.

Helping a client transfer using a slide board

1. Follow steps 1 through 9 of the procedure for transferring a client from a bed to a wheelchair or chair.

2. Have the client lean away from transfer side to take the weight off her thigh (Fig. 4-11). Place one end of the sliding board under the buttocks and thigh. Take care not to pinch the client's skin between the bed and the board. Place the other end of the sliding board on the surface to which the client is transferring.

3. If the client is able, have her push up with her hands and scoot herself across the board. Stay close so you can provide support if needed. Always allow the client to do all she can for herself.

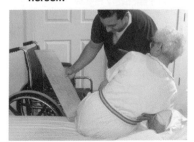

Fig. 4-11. While placing the transfer board, be careful not to pinch the skin between the bed and the board.

4. If the client needs assistance, stand in front of her and put your knees in front and a little to the outside of her knees to keep them from buckling during the transfer. Make sure your back is straight.

5. Get as close to the client as possible and have her lean into you as you grasp the transfer belt from behind. Lean back with your knees bent. Using your legs rather than your back, pull the client up slightly and toward you to help her scoot across the board (Fig. 4-12).

6. Complete the transfer in two or three lifting and scooting movements. Never drag the client across the board. Friction from the client's skin dragging across the slide board can cause skin breakdown that can lead to pressure sores.

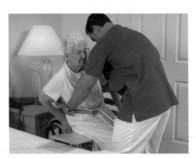

Fig. 4-12. Help the client scoot across board while keeping your knees slightly bent.

7. After the client is safely transferred, remove the slide board. Make sure the client is positioned safely and comfortably.

8. Wash your hands.

9. Document the procedure and any observations. How did the client feel or appear during the transfer? How much assistance was required?

You may assist the client with many types of transfers using a mechanical, or hydraulic, lift if you are trained to do so. Lifts help prevent injury to you and the client. Never use equipment you have not been trained to use. You or your client could get hurt if you use lifting equipment improperly. There are many different types of mechanical lifts. You must be trained on the specific lift you will be using. Ask someone to help you before starting.

Transferring a client using a mechanical lift

Equipment: wheelchair or chair, lifting partner (if available), mechanical or hydraulic lift

1. Wash your hands.

2. Explain the procedure to the client, speaking clearly, slowly, and directly. Maintain face-to-face contact whenever possible.

3. Provide privacy if the client desires it.

4. If bed is movable, lock bed wheels.

5. Position wheelchair near bed. Lock brakes.

6. Help the client turn to one side of the bed. Position the sling under the client, with the edge next to the client's back fanfolded if necessary, and the bottom of the sling even with

the client's knees. Help the client roll back to the middle of the bed, and then spread out the fanfolded edge of the sling.

7. Roll the mechanical lift to bedside. Make sure the base is opened to its widest point, and push the base of the lift under the bed.

8. Position the overhead bar directly over the client (Fig. 4-13).

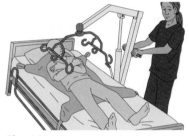

Fig. 4-13.

9. With the client lying on his back, attach one set of straps to each side of the sling, and one set of straps to the overhead bar (Fig. 4-14). If available, have a lifting partner support the client at the head and shoulders and at the knees while the client is being lifted. The client's arms should be folded across her chest. If the device has "S" hooks, they should face away from client.

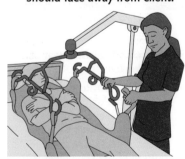

Fig. 4-14.

10. Following manufacturer's instructions for operating the lift, raise the client two inches above the bed. Pause a moment for the client to gain balance.

11. If available, a lifting partner can help support and guide the client's body while you roll the lift so that the client is positioned over the chair or wheelchair (Fig. 4-15).

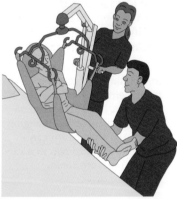

Fig. 4-15.

12. Slowly lower the client into the chair or wheelchair. Push down gently on the client's knees to help the client into a sitting, rather than reclining, position.

13. Undo the straps from the overhead bar to the sling. Leave the sling in place for transfer back to bed.

14. Be sure the client is seated comfortably and correctly in the chair or wheelchair.

15. Wash your hands.

16. Document the procedure and any observations. How did the client tolerate the transfer? Were there any problems? Did the equipment operate properly?

Ambulation is walking. A client who is **ambulatory** is one who can get out of bed and walk. Many older clients are ambulatory, but need assistance to walk safely. Several tools, including gait belts, canes, walkers, and crutches, assist with ambulation.

Assisting a client to ambulate

Equipment: gait belt, non-skid shoes for the client

1. Wash your hands.

2. Explain the procedure to the client, speaking clearly, slowly, and directly. Maintain face-to-face contact whenever possible.

3. Provide privacy if the client desires it.

4. Before ambulating, put on and properly fasten non-skid footwear on client.

5. If the bed is adjustable, adjust bed to a low position. Lock bed wheels. Assist client to sitting position with feet flat on the floor.

6. Stand in front of and face the client.

7. With your legs, brace client's lower legs to prevent slipping. This can be done by placing both of your knees in front of the client's knees. It can also be done by placing both of your knees on the outside of both of the client's legs. Follow agency policy.

8. *With gait (transfer) belt*: Place belt around client's waist over clothing (not on bare skin). Bend your knees and lean forward. Grasp the belt on both sides. Hold him close to your center of gravity. Tell the client to lean forward, push down on the bed with her hands, and stand, on the count of three. When you start to count, begin to rock. At three, rock your weight onto your back foot. Assist client to a standing position.

Without gait belt: Place arms around client's torso under armpits, while assisting client to stand.

9. *With gait belt*: Walk slightly behind and to one side of client for the full distance, while holding onto the gait belt (Fig. 4-16).

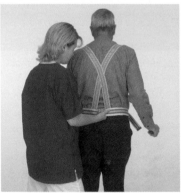

Fig. 4-16. Walk behind and to one side while holding onto the gait belt when assisting with ambulation.

Without gait belt: Walk slightly behind and to one side of client for the full distance. Support client's back with your arm. If the client has a weaker side, stand on that side. Use the hand that is not holding the belt or the arm not on the back to offer support on the weak side.

10. After ambulation, remove gait belt if used. Help client to the bed or chair and make client comfortable. If you raised an adjustable bed, return it to its lowest position.

11. Wash your hands.

12. Document the procedure and your observations. How far did the client walk? How did the client appear or say he felt while walking? How much help did you give?

Clients who have difficulty walking may use adaptive devices, such as canes, walkers, or crutches to help themselves. When assisting with these devices, remember the following:

- Make sure the equipment is in proper condition. It must be sturdy, and it must have rubber tips or wheels on the bottom.
- Be sure the client is wearing non-skid shoes that are securely fastened.
- When using a cane, the client should place it on his stronger side.
- When using a walker, have the client place both hands on the walker. The walker should not be over-extended. It should be placed no more than 12 inches in front of the client.
- Stay near the client, on the weak side.

Assisting with ambulation for a client who uses a cane, walker, or crutches

Equipment: gait belt, non-skid shoes for client, cane, walker, or crutches

1. Wash your hands.

2. Explain the procedure to the client, speaking clearly, slowly, and directly. Maintain face-to-face contact whenever possible.

3. Provide privacy if the client desires it.

4. Before ambulating, put on and properly fasten non-skid footwear on client.

5. If the bed is adjustable, adjust bed to low position so that the feet are flat on the floor. If the bed is movable, lock bed wheels. Assist client to sitting position with feet flat on the floor.

6. Stand in front of and face the client.

7. With your legs, brace client's lower legs to prevent slipping. This can be done by placing both of your knees in front of the client's knees. It can also be done by placing both of your knees on the outside of both of the client's legs. Follow agency policy.

8. Place the gait belt around the client's waist over clothing (not on bare skin). Grasp the belt on both sides while helping the client to stand as previously described.

9. Assist as needed with ambulation.

a. *Cane:* Client places cane about 12 inches in front of his stronger leg. He brings weaker leg even with cane. He then brings stronger leg forward slightly ahead of cane (Fig. 4-17). Repeat.

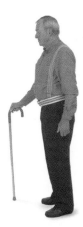

Fig. 4-17. *The cane moves in front of the stronger leg first.*

b. *Walker*: Client picks up or rolls the walker and places it about 12 inches in front of him. All four feet or wheels of the walker should be on the ground before client steps forward to the walker. The walker should not be moved again until the client has moved both feet forward and is steady (Fig. 4-18). The client should never put his feet ahead of the walker.

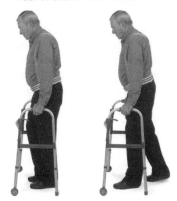

Fig. 4-18. *The walker can be moved after the client is steady and both feet are forward.*

c. *Crutches*: Client should be fitted for crutches and taught to use them correctly by a physical therapist or a nurse. The client may use the crutches several different ways. No matter how they are used, the client's weight should be on his hands and arms. Weight should not be on the underarm area (Fig. 4-19).

10. Whether the client is using a cane, walker, or crutches, walk slightly behind and to one side of client. Stay on the weak side if the client has one. Hold the gait belt if one is used.

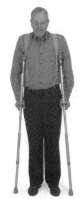

Fig. 4-19. *When using crutches, weight should be on the hands and arms, not on the underarms.*

11. Watch for obstacles in the client's path. Ask the client to look ahead, not down at his feet.

12. Encourage the client to rest if tired. Allowing a client to become too tired increases the chance of a fall. Let the client set the pace. Discuss how far he plans to go based on the care plan.

13. After ambulation, remove the gait belt. Settle the client back into a safe and comfortable position after ambulation. If you raised an adjustable bed, return it to its lowest position.

14. Wash your hands.

15. Document the procedure and your observations. How did the client feel or appear while walking? How far did the client walk? How much help did the client need?

Range of Motion Exercises

Exercise helps people regain strength and mobility. It prevents disabilities from developing. People who are in bed for long periods of time are more likely to develop contractures. A contracture is the permanent and often very painful stiffening of a joint and muscle. Contractures are generally caused by immobility and result in a loss of ability. **Range of motion (ROM)** exercises are exercises that put a joint through its full arc of motion. The goal of ROM exercises is to decrease or prevent contractures, improve strength, and increase circulation.

Passive range of motion (PROM) exercises are used when clients cannot move on their own. When assisting with PROM exercises, support the client's joints. Move them through the range of motion. Active assisted range of motion (AAROM) exercises are performed by the client with some help and support from you. Active range of motion (AROM) exercises are performed by a client himself. Your role in AROM exercises is to encourage the client.

You will not perform ROM exercises without an order from a doctor, nurse, or physical therapist. When performing ROM exercises, begin at the client's head and work down the body. Exercise the upper extremities (arms) before the lower extremities (legs). Give support above and below the joint. Stop the motion if the client complains of pain. These exercises are specific for each body area. They include these movements (Fig. 4-20):

- **Abduction**: moving a body part away from the midline of the body
- **Adduction**: moving a body part toward the midline of the body
- **Dorsiflexion**: bending backward
- **Rotation**: turning a joint
- **Extension**: straightening a body part
- **Flexion**: bending a body part
- **Pronation**: turning downward
- **Supination**: turning upward

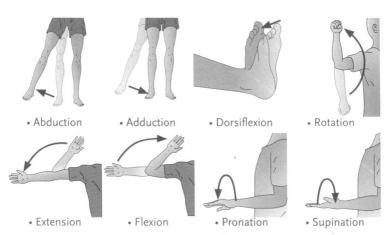

- Abduction   • Adduction   • Dorsiflexion   • Rotation

- Extension   • Flexion   • Pronation   • Supination

Fig. 4-20. Different range of motion body movements.

Assisting with passive range of motion exercises

1. Wash your hands.

2. Explain the procedure to the client, speaking clearly, slowly, and directly. Maintain face-to-face contact whenever possible.

3. Provide privacy if the client desires it.

4. If the bed is adjustable, adjust bed a safe level, usually waist high. If the bed is movable, lock bed wheels.

5. Position the client lying supine—flat on his or her back—on the bed. Position body in good alignment.

6. Repeat each exercise at least three times. While supporting the limbs, move all joints gently, slowly, and smoothly through the range of motion to the point of resistance. Stop if any pain occurs.

7. *Shoulder.* Support client's arm at elbow and wrist while performing ROM for the shoulder. Place one hand under the elbow and the other hand under the wrist. Raise the straightened arm from the side

position forward to above the head and return arm to side of the body (flexion/extension) (Fig. 4-21).

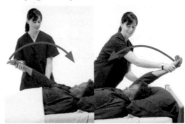

Fig. 4-21.

Raise the arm to side position above head and return arm to side of the body (abduction/adduction) (Fig. 4-22).

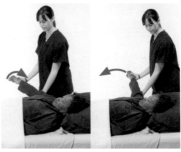

Fig. 4-22.

8. *Elbow.* Hold the wrist with one hand. Hold the elbow with the other hand. Bend elbow so that the hand touches the shoulder on that same side (flexion). Straighten arm (extension) (Fig. 4-23).

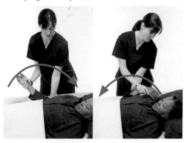

Fig. 4-23.

Exercise forearm by moving it so palm is facing downward (pronation) and then upward (supination) (Fig. 4-24).

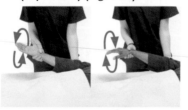

Fig. 4-24.

9. *Wrist.* Hold the wrist with one hand. Use the fingers of the other hand to help the joint through the motions. Bend the hand down (flexion). Bend the hand backwards (extension) (Fig. 4-25).

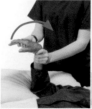

Fig. 4-25.

Turn the hand in the direction of the thumb (radial flexion). Then turn the hand in the direction of the little finger (ulnar flexion) (Fig. 4-26).

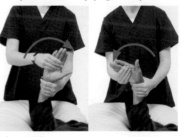

Fig. 4-26.

10. *Thumb.* Move the thumb away from the index finger (abduction). Move the thumb back next to the index finger (adduction) (Fig. 4-27).

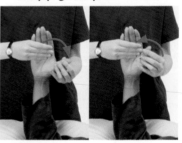

Fig. 4-27.

Touch each fingertip with the thumb (opposition) (Fig. 4-28).

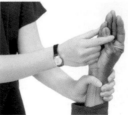

Fig. 4-28.

Bend thumb into the palm (flexion) and out to the side (extension) (Fig. 4-29).

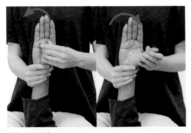

Fig. 4-29.

11. *Fingers.* Make the hand into a fist (flexion). Gently straighten out the fist (extension) (Fig. 4-30).

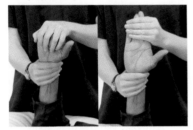

Fig. 4-30.

Spread the fingers and the thumb far apart from each other (abduction). Bring the fingers back next to each other (adduction) (Fig. 4-31).

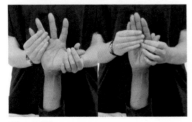

Fig. 4-31.

12. *Hip.* Support the leg by placing one hand under the knee and one under the ankle. Straighten the leg. Raise it gently upward. Move the leg away from the other leg (abduction). Move the leg toward the other leg (adduction) (Fig. 4-32).

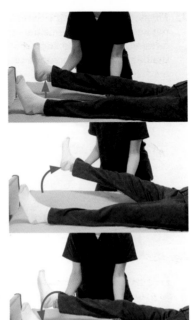

Fig. 4-32.

Gently turn the leg inward (internal rotation). Turn the leg outward (external rotation) (Fig. 4-33).

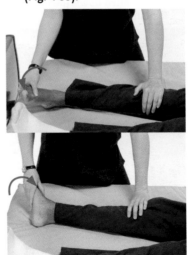

Fig. 4-33.

13. *Knees.* Support the leg under the knee and ankle while performing ROM for the knee. Bend the leg to the point of resistance (flexion). Return leg to client's normal position (extension) (Fig. 4-34).

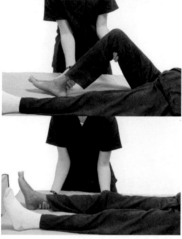

Fig. 4-34.

14. *Ankles.* Push/pull foot up toward head (dorsiflexion). Push/pull foot down, with the toes pointed down (plantar flexion) (Fig. 4-35).

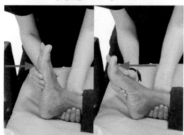

Fig. 4-35.

Turn inside of the foot inward toward the body (supination). Bend the sole of the foot away from the body (pronation) (Fig. 4-36).

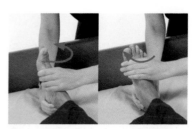

Fig. 4-36.

15. *Toes.* Curl and straighten the toes (flexion and extension) (Fig. 4-37).

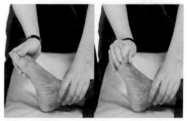

Fig. 4-37.

Gently spread the toes apart (abduction) (Fig. 4-38).

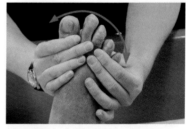

Fig. 4-38.

16. Return client to comfortable position.

17. Wash your hands.

18. Document the procedure. Note any decrease in range of motion or any pain experienced by the client. Notify the supervisor or the physical therapist if you find increased stiffness or physical resistance. Resistance may be a sign that a contracture is developing.

Skin Care

Clients who have restricted mobility have greater risk of skin deterioration at pressure points. Pressure points are areas of the body that bear much of the body weight. Pressure points are mainly located at bony prominences. Bony prominences are areas of the body where the bone lies close to the skin. These areas include elbows, shoulder blades, tailbone, hip bones, ankles, heels, and the back of the neck and head. The skin here is at a much higher risk for skin breakdown.

Other areas at risk are the ears, the area under the breasts, and the scrotum (Fig. 4-39). The pressure on these areas reduces circulation, decreasing the amount of oxygen the cells receive. Warmth and moisture also add to skin breakdown. Once the surface of the skin is weakened, pathogens can invade and cause infection. When infection occurs, the healing process slows.

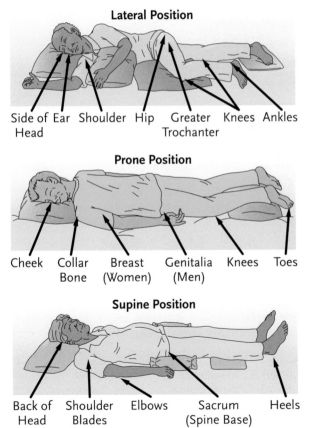

Lateral Position

Side of Head · Ear · Shoulder · Hip · Greater Trochanter · Knees · Ankles

Prone Position

Cheek · Collar Bone · Breast (Women) · Genitalia (Men) · Knees · Toes

Supine Position

Back of Head · Shoulder Blades · Elbows · Sacrum (Spine Base) · Heels

Fig. 4-39. Pressure sore danger zones.

When the skin begins to break down, it becomes pale, white or a red-dened color. Darker skin may look purple. The client may also feel tingling or burning in the area. This discoloration does not go away, even when the client's position is changed. If pressure is allowed to continue, the area will further break down. The resulting wound is called a **pressure sore**, pressure ulcer, bed sore, or decubitus ulcer. Once a pressure sore forms, it can get bigger, deeper, and infected. Pressure sores are painful and are difficult to heal. They can lead to life-threatening infections. Prevention is the key to skin health.

Observing and Reporting: Client's Skin

O/R Pale, white, reddened, or purple areas

O/R Blisters or bruises on the skin

O/R Complaints of tingling, warmth, or burning of the skin

O/R Dry or flaking skin

O/R Itching or scratching

O/R Rash or any skin discoloration

O/R Swelling

O/R Fluid or blood draining from skin

O/R Broken skin

O/R Wounds or ulcers on the skin

O/R Changes in wound or ulcer (size, depth, drainage, color, odor)

O/R Redness or broken skin between toes or around toenails

In darker complexions, also look for

O/R Any change in the feel of the tissue, any change in the appearance of the skin, such as the "orange-peel" look or a purplish hue, and extremely dry, crust-like areas that might be covering a tissue break

---

Guidelines: Basic Skin Care

G Report changes you observe in a client's skin.

G Provide regular, daily care for skin to keep it clean and dry. Always check the client's skin when bathing.

G Reposition immobile clients often (at least every two hours).

G Give frequent and thorough skin care as often as needed for incontinent clients. Change clothing and linens often as well.

G Do not scratch or irritate the skin in any way. Keep rough, scratchy fabrics away from the client's skin. Report to your supervisor if a client wears shoes or slippers that cause blisters or sores.

G Massage the skin often. Use light, circular strokes to increase circulation. Use little or no pressure on bony areas. Do not massage a white, red, or purple area or put any pressure on it. Massage the healthy skin and tissue surrounding the area.

G Be careful during transfers. Avoid pulling or tearing fragile skin.

G Clients who are overweight may have poor circulation and extra folds of skin. Pay careful attention to the skin under the folds. Keep it clean and dry. Report signs of skin irritation.

G Encourage well-balanced meals. Proper nutrition is important for keeping skin healthy.

G Keep plastic or rubber materials from coming into contact with the client's skin. These materials prevent air from circulating, which causes the skin to sweat.

G The skin may have to be washed with a special soap, or a brush may have to be used on the skin. Follow the care plan and ask your supervisor if you have any questions.

For clients who are confined to bed, remember:

G Keep the bottom sheet tight and free from wrinkles and the bed free from crumbs. Keep clothing or gowns free of wrinkles, too.

G Do not pull the client across sheets during transfers or repositioning. This can cause **shearing**, which can lead to skin breakdown.

G Place a sheepskin, chamois skin, or bed pad under the back and buttocks to absorb moisture. This also protects the skin from irritating bed linens.

G Relieve pressure under bony prominences. Place foam rubber or sheepskin pads under them. Heel and elbow protectors that are made of foam and sheepskin are available.

G A bed or chair can be made softer with flotation pads.

G Use a bed cradle to keep top sheets from rubbing the client's skin.

G Reposition clients seated in chairs or wheelchairs often.

Comfort Measures

There are several things you can do to provide for the comfort and safety of your client in and around the bed. Many positioning devices are available to help make clients more comfortable. Some can be inexpensively made in the client's home. Check with your supervisor about the use of positioning devices for each client.

Guidelines: Positioning Devices

G Backrests provide support. They can be made of pillows, cardboard or wood covered by pillows, or special wedge-shaped foam pillows.

G Bed cradles are used to keep the bed covers from pushing down on client's feet. Metal frames that work like a tent when the bed covers are over them can be purchased. A cardboard box can be used as a bed cradle by placing the client's feet inside the box underneath the covers. The box should be at least two inches above the toes.

G Bed tables are available commercially. You can also make one by cutting openings in each of the longer sides of a sturdy cardboard box.

G Draw sheets may be placed under a client to help move clients who are unable to assist with turning in bed, lifting, or moving up in bed. Draw sheets also help prevent skin damage that can be caused by shearing. A regular bed sheet folded in half can be used as a draw sheet.

G Foot boards are padded boards placed against the client's feet to keep them properly aligned and to prevent **foot drop**. Rolled blankets or pillows can also be used as foot boards.

G Hand rolls keep the fingers from curling tightly. A rolled washcloth, gauze bandage, or a rubber ball placed inside the palm may be used to keep the hand in a natural position.

G Splints may be prescribed by a doctor to keep a client's joints in the correct position. Splints are a type of orthotic device. An **orthotic device** is a device, such as a splint or brace, that helps support and align a limb and improve its functioning. Orthotics also help prevent or correct deformities. Splints and the skin area around them should be cleaned at least once daily and as needed.

G Trochanter rolls are used to keep the client's hips from turning outward. A rolled towel works well as a trochanter roll.

G Knee pillows, or regular pillows placed between the knees, can help keep spine, hips, and knees in the proper position and ease pain in the back, leg, hip and knee areas.

A back rub can help relax your client and make her more comfortable. Back rubs increase circulation, too. Back rubs are often given after baths.

Giving a back rub

Equipment: cotton blanket or towel, lotion

1. Wash your hands.

2. **Explain the procedure to the client, speaking clearly, slowly, and directly. Maintain face-to-face contact whenever possible.**

3. Provide privacy if the client desires it.

4. If the bed is adjustable, adjust bed to a safe working level, usually waist high. Lower the head of the bed. If the bed is movable, lock bed wheels.

5. Have the client lie in a prone position. If this is uncomfortable, have the client lie on his side (Fig. 4-40). Cover the client with a cotton blanket, then fold back the bed covers. Expose the client's back to the top of the buttocks. Back rubs can also be given with the client sitting up.

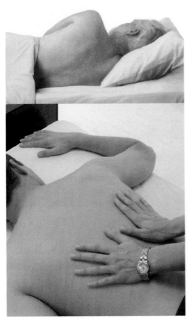

Fig. 4-40. A client can be on his side or on his stomach for back rubs.

6. Warm the lotion bottle in warm water for five minutes. Run your hands under warm water to warm them. Pour the lotion on your hands. Rub them together to spread it. Warn the client that the lotion may still feel cool. Always put the lotion on your hands rather than directly on the client's skin.

7. Place your hands on each side of the upper part of the buttocks. Make long, smooth upward strokes with both hands along each side of the spine, up to the shoulders. Circle your hands outward. Then move back along the outer edges of the back. At the buttocks, make another circle and move your hands back up to the shoulders. Without taking your hands from the client's skin, repeat this motion for three to five minutes.

8. Make kneading motions with the first two fingers and thumb of each hand. Place them at the base of the spine. Move upward together along each side of the spine, applying gentle downward pressure with the fingers and thumbs. Follow the same direction as with the long smooth strokes, circling at shoulders and buttocks.

9. Gently massage bony areas (spine, shoulder blades, hip bones) with circular motions of your fingertips. Gentle massage stimulates circulation and helps prevent skin damage. However, if any of these areas are red, massage around them rather than on them. The redness indicates that the skin is already irritated and fragile.

10. Let your client know when you are almost through. Finish with some long smooth strokes, like the ones you used at the beginning of the massage.

11. Dry the back if extra lotion remains on it. If appropriate, apply powder to the back to allow better movement against the sheets.

12. Remove the cotton blanket and towel.

13. Assist the client with getting dressed.

14. Help the client into a comfortable position. If you raised an adjustable bed, return it to its lowest position.

15. Store the lotion and put dirty linens in the hamper.

16. Wash your hands.

17. Document the procedure and your observations. Did the client appear comfortable during the back rub? Did you observe any discolored areas or broken skin?

Personal Care Procedures

If you are already a CNA or HHA, you have previously learned personal care skills. This section will serve as a review of the basic skills and procedures most often provided for clients in their homes. Clients should be encouraged to do as much of the care by themselves as possible. This promotes independence.

Hygiene is the term used to describe ways to keep bodies clean and healthy. Bathing and brushing teeth are two examples. Grooming refers to practices like caring for fingernails and hair. Hygiene and grooming activities, as well as dressing, eating, transferring, and toileting are called **activities of daily living (ADLs)**. Personal care includes such activities as bathing, perineal care (care of the genital and anal area), toileting, mouth care, shampooing and combing the hair, nail care, shaving, dressing, eating, walking, transferring, and changing bed linens.

Before you begin any task, explain to the client exactly what you will be doing. Explaining care to a client is not only his legal right, but it may also help lessen anxiety. Ask if he or she would like to use the bathroom or bedpan first. Provide the client with privacy. Let him or her make as many decisions as possible about when, where, and how a procedure will be done. This promotes dignity and independence. During the procedure, if the client appears tired, stop and take a short rest. After care, always ask if the client would like anything else.

Observing and Reporting: Personal Care

%r   Skin color, temperature, redness

%r   Mobility

^o/_R   Flexibility

^o/_R   Comfort level, or complaints of pain or discomfort

^o/_R   Strength and the ability to perform self-care and ADLs

^o/_R   Mental and emotional state

^o/_R   Client complaints

Bathing

Bathing promotes good health and well-being. It removes perspiration, dirt, oil, and dead skin cells that collect on the skin. Taking a bath or having a bed bath can also be relaxing. The bed bath is an excellent time for moving arms and legs and increasing circulation. Many agencies have rules against HHAs helping clients into the bathtub. These rules are for the client's safety as well as the home health aide's. Follow your agency's policies and procedures. Some clients may be embarrassed or uncomfortable with someone helping them bathe. Be sensitive to this. Provide privacy, and be professional and respectful.

Guidelines: Bathing

G   The face, hands, axillae (underarms), and perineum should be washed every day. A complete bath or shower can be taken every other day or even less frequently. Older skin produces less perspiration and oil. Elderly people whose skin is dry and fragile should bathe only once or twice a week. Be gentle with the skin when bathing older clients.

G   Before any bathing task, make sure the room is warm enough.

G   Remove any loose rugs that do not have slip-resistant, rubber backings.

G   Be familiar with available safety and assistive devices.

G   Before bathing, make sure the water temperature is safe and comfortable. Test the water temperature to make sure it is not too hot. Then have the client test the water temperature. The client is best able to choose a comfortable water temperature.

G   Never leave an elderly person or young child alone in the bathtub. Gather supplies before giving a bath so the client is not left alone.

G   Make sure all soap is removed from the skin before completing the bath.

G   Do not use bath oils, lotions, or powders in showers or tubs. They make surfaces slippery.

You may have to adapt this procedure to work with your clients' different strength levels.

Helping a client transfer to the bathtub

Equipment: chair or wheelchair, transfer belt (if appropriate), shirt or robe to wear under transfer belt, slide board (if appropriate), tub or shower chair, bath supplies (as listed in next procedure)

1. Wash your hands.

2. Explain the procedure to the client, speaking clearly, slowly, and directly. Maintain face-to-face contact whenever possible.

3. Help the client to the bath-room.

4. Provide privacy for the client.

5. Seat the client in a chair facing the bathtub and centered between the grab bars. If using a wheelchair, lock brakes and raise footrests (Fig. 4-41).

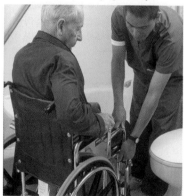

Fig. 4-41. Lock the wheelchair before beginning to transfer a client.

6. Ask the client to place one leg at a time over the sides of the tub.

7. Have client hold on to the grab bars or the edge of the tub to bring himself to a sitting position on the edge of the tub

(Fig. 4-42). A slide board may also be used to help the client move from the chair to the tub

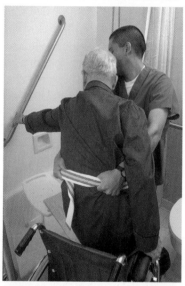

Fig. 4-42. Have client hold onto grab bars while moving him into the tub. Keep your back straight and your knees slightly bent while assisting with the move.

8. Help the client lower himself into the tub or onto the tub chair (bath bench) while holding on to the edge of the tub or grab bars. If necessary, assist by holding him around the waist or by having him wear a transfer belt. If using a transfer belt to get in and out of the tub, the client will need to wear a shirt or robe while transferring, so the belt is not placed directly against his skin. When he is in the tub, place supplies within easy reach (Fig. 4-43).

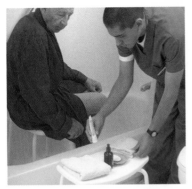

Fig. 4-43. Keep bathing supplies close to client during shower or tub bath.

9. Reverse this procedure to help the client out of the tub when the bath is over. If the client has trouble getting out of the tub, help him to his hands and knees. From that position, he can use the grab bar or the edge of the tub to help pull himself up. You can also help by putting the transfer belt back on the client (over a robe).

10. Wash your hands.

11. Document the procedure and your observations.

Clients who can get out of bed to take a shower or bath will need different assistance and supervision. Follow the instructions in the care plan.

Helping the ambulatory client take a shower or tub bath

Equipment: two bath towels, washcloth, soap or other cleanser, bath thermometer (if available), rubber bath mat, tub or shower chair (if appropriate), table for bath supplies and bell (for clients who bathe without assistance), non-skid bath rug, deodorant, lotion and other toiletries, clean clothes or a robe, shoes or non-skid slippers, gloves

1. Wash your hands.

2. Explain the procedure to the client, speaking clearly, slowly, and directly. Maintain face-to-face contact whenever possible.

3. Clean tub or shower if necessary. Place rubber mat on tub or shower floor. Set up tub or shower chair. Place non-skid bath rug on the floor next to the tub or shower.

4. Provide privacy for the client.

5. Put on gloves.

6. Fill the tub with warm water (105° to 110°F on the bath ther-

mometer, or test the water on the inside of your wrist to see if it is comfortable) or adjust the shower water temperature.

Have the client test water temperature to see if it is comfortable. Adjust if necessary.

7. Ask the client to undress, and assist as needed. Help client transfer to bathtub or step in the shower.

8. If the care plan allows you to leave the client to bathe alone, place the bathing supplies on a small table within the client's reach. Place a bell or other signal on the table (Fig. 4-44). Tell the client to signal when you are needed. Ask the client not to add more hot or warm water and not to remain in the tub more than 20 minutes. Do not lock the bathroom door. Check on your client every five minutes. If the client is weak, remain in the bathroom. Otherwise, you can make the

client's bed while he is in the tub.

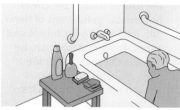

Fig. 4-44. A bell or other signal provides a way for the client to communicate that he needs you.

9. For a shower, stay with the client and assist with washing hard-to-reach areas. Observe for signs of fatigue.

10. If the client needs more assistance in the bath or shower, help him wash himself. Always wash from clean areas to dirty areas, so you do not spread dirt into areas that have already been washed. Make sure all soap is rinsed off so the client's skin does not become dry or irritated.

11. Assist the client with shampooing hair, if necessary (see procedure later in chapter). Make sure all shampoo is rinsed out of hair.

12. When the bath or shower is finished, help the client get out of the tub. Wrap him in a towel. Have the client sit in a chair or on the toilet seat, and provide him with another towel for drying himself (Fig. 4-45). Offer

assistance in drying hard-to-reach places. The client may need help applying powder, deodorant, or lotion. If necessary, help the client get dressed.

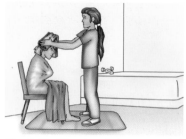

Fig. 4-45. Give the client any needed assistance when drying herself.

13. If your client is tired after the bath or shower, help him back to the bed. Other personal care, such as mouth care, can be done later or while the client is in bed.

14. Clean the tub and place soiled laundry (towels, washcloths, dirty clothes) in the hamper. Remove and discard gloves.

15. Wash your hands.

16. Put away supplies.

17. Document the procedure and your observations. Did you observe any redness or whiteness on the skin? Was there any broken skin? How did the client tolerate bathing or showering? Has there been a change in the client's abilities since the last bath or shower?

Giving a complete bed bath

Equipment: soft cotton blanket or large towel, bath basin, soap, bath thermometer (if available), 2-4 washcloths, 2-4 towels, clean gown or clothes, gloves, lotion, deodorant, orangewood stick or nail brush (if available)

1. Wash your hands.

2. Explain the procedure to the client, speaking clearly, slowly, and directly. Maintain face-to-face contact whenever possible.

3. Provide privacy for the client. Be sure the room is a comfortable temperature and there are no drafts.

4. If the bed is adjustable, adjust bed to a safe working level, usually waist high. If the bed is movable, lock bed wheels.

5. Ask client to remove glasses and jewelry and put them in a safe place. Offer a bedpan or urinal for the client to use before the bath.

6. Place a soft cotton blanket or towel over client (Fig. 4-46), and ask him to hold on to it as you remove or fold back top bedding. Remove gown, while keeping client covered with blanket (or top sheet). Check the sheets for spills or body discharges.

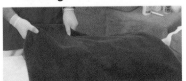

Fig. 4-46. *Cover the client with a cotton blanket before removing top bedding.*

7. Fill the basin with warm water. Test water temperature with a bath thermometer or against the inside of your wrist. Water temperature should be between 105° and 110°F. It cools quickly. Have the client test water temperature to see if it is comfortable. Adjust if necessary. During the bath, change the water when it becomes too cool, soapy, or dirty.

8. Put on gloves.

9. Ask and assist the client to participate in washing.

10. Uncover only one part of the body at a time. Place a towel under the body part being washed.

11. Wash, rinse, and dry one part of the body at a time. Start at the head. Work down, and complete the front first. When washing, use a clean area of the washcloth for each stroke.

Eyes and Face: Wash face with wet washcloth (no soap). Begin with the eye farther away from you. Wash inner aspect to outer aspect (Fig. 4-47). Use a different area of the washcloth for each eye. Wash the face from the middle outward. Use firm but gentle strokes. Wash the neck and ears and behind the ears. Rinse and pat dry.

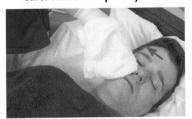

Fig. 4-47. *Wash the eye from the inner part to the outer part.*

Arms: Remove one arm from under the towel. With a soapy washcloth, wash the upper arm and underarm. Use long strokes from the shoulder to the wrist (Fig. 4-48). Rinse and pat dry. Repeat for the other arm.

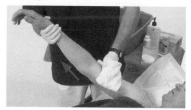

Fig. 4-48. Support the wrist while washing the shoulder, arm, underarm, and elbow.

Hands: Wash one hand in a basin. Clean under the nails with an orangewood stick or nail brush (Fig. 4-49). Rinse and pat dry. Give nail care if it has been assigned (see procedure later in this chapter). Repeat for the other hand. Put lotion on the client's elbows and hands if ordered.

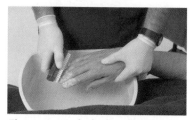

Fig. 4-49. Wash the hand in a basin. Thoroughly clean under the nails with a nail brush.

Chest: Place the towel across the client's chest. Pull the blanket down to the waist. Lift the towel only enough to wash the chest. Rinse it and pat dry. For a female client, wash, rinse, and dry breasts and under breasts. Check the skin in this area for signs of irritation.

Abdomen: Keep towel across chest. Fold the blanket down so that it still covers the pubic

area. Wash the abdomen, rinse, and pat dry. If the client has an ostomy, give skin care around the opening (see "Special Procedures" section). Cover with the towel. Pull the cotton blanket up to the client's chin. Remove the towel.

Legs and Feet: Expose one leg. Place a towel under it. Wash the thigh. Use long downward strokes. Rinse and pat dry. Do the same from the knee to the ankle (Fig. 4-50).

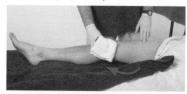

Fig. 4-50. Use long downward strokes when washing the legs.

Place another towel under the foot. Move the basin to the towel. Place the foot into the basin. Wash the foot and between the toes (Fig. 4-51). Rinse foot and pat dry. Make sure area between toes is dry. Give nail care if it has been assigned. Do not give nail care to a diabetic client. Never clip a client's toenails. Apply lotion to the foot if ordered, especially at the heels. Do not apply lotion between the toes. Repeat steps for the other leg and foot.

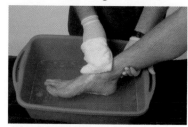

Fig. 4-51. Wash the feet and between the toes.

Back: Help client move to the center of the bed. Ask client to turn onto his side so his back is facing you. If the bed has rails, raise the rail on the far side for safety. Fold the blanket away from the back. Place a towel lengthwise next to the back. Wash the neck and back with long, downward strokes (Fig. 4-52). Rinse and pat dry. Apply lotion if ordered.

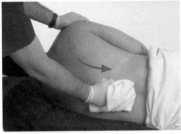

Fig. 4-52. Wash the back with long, downward strokes.

12. Place the towel under the buttocks and upper thighs. Help the client turn onto his back. If the client is able to wash his or her perineal area, place a basin of clean, warm water and a washcloth and towel within reach. Hand items to the client as needed. If the client wants you to leave the room, leave supplies within reach. If the client has a urinary catheter in place, remind him or her not to pull it.

13. If the client cannot provide perineal care, you must do so. Provide privacy at all times.

Perineal area: Change bath water. Put on clean gloves. Wash, rinse, and dry perineal area. Work from front to back.

For a female client: Wash the perineum with soap and water. Work from front to back. Use single strokes (Fig. 4-53). Do not wash from the back to the front. This may cause infection. Use a clean area of washcloth or clean washcloth for each stroke. First wipe the center of the perineum, then each side. Then spread the labia majora, the outside folds of perineal skin that protect the urinary meatus and the vaginal opening. Wipe from front to back on each side. Rinse the area in the same way. Dry entire perineal area. Move from front to back. Use a blotting motion with towel. Ask client to turn on her side. Wash, rinse, and dry buttocks and anal area. Clean the anal area without contaminating the perineal area.

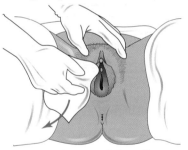

Fig. 4-53. Always work from front to back when performing perineal care. This helps prevent infection.

For a male client: If the client is uncircumcised, pull back the foreskin first. Gently push skin towards the base of penis. Hold the penis by the shaft. Wash in a circular motion from the tip down to the base. Use a clean area of washcloth or clean washcloth for each stroke (Fig. 4-54). Rinse the penis. If client is uncircumcised, gently return foreskin to normal position. Then wash the scrotum and groin. The groin is the area from the pubis (area around the penis and scrotum) to the upper thighs. Rinse and pat dry. Ask the client to turn on his side. Wash, rinse, and dry buttocks and anal area. Clean the anal area without contaminating the perineal area.

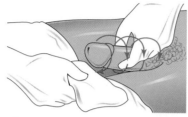

Fig. 4-54.

14. Cover the client with the cotton blanket.

15. Place soiled washcloths and towels in the hamper or laundry basket. Dispose of the dirty bath water in the toilet.

16. Remove and discard gloves. Wash your hands.

17. If time permits, a bed bath is a good time to give the client a back rub if he wants one.

18. Provide the client with deodorant. Place a towel over the pillow and brush or comb the client's hair (see procedure later in this chapter). Help the client put on clean clothing and get into a comfortable position with good body alignment. If you raised an adjustable bed, return it to its lowest position.

19. If the client uses a signaling device, place it within reach. Take the bath supplies away, and wash and store everything. Change bed sheets and blanket. Place used bed linens in the hamper or laundry basket.

20. Wash your hands.

21. Document the procedure and your observations. Did you observe any redness, whiteness, or purple areas on the skin? Was there any broken skin? How did the client tolerate bathing? Did the client tell you about any symptoms? Has there been a change in the client's abilities since the last bath?

Grooming

When assisting clients with grooming, always let clients to do all they can for themselves. Follow the instructions in the care plan. Some clients have particular ways of grooming themselves. They may have routines. Some clients may be embarrassed or depressed because they need help with grooming tasks they have performed for themselves all their lives. Be sensitive to this. Be professional, respectful and cheerful while assisting your clients with grooming.

Clients who can get out of bed may have their hair shampooed in the sink, tub, or shower. For clients who cannot get out of bed, special troughs exist for shampooing hair in bed. Troughs fit under the client's head and neck and have a spout or hose that drains the water into a basin at the side of the bed. Your agency should be able to provide this equipment. You may also use a plastic garbage bag formed around a rolled towel.

Shampooing hair

Equipment: shampoo, hair conditioner (if requested), 2 bath towels, washcloth, pitcher or hand-held shower or sink attachment, plastic cup, waterproof pad (for washing hair in bed), cotton blanket (for washing hair in bed), trough or garbage bag and extra towel (for washing hair in bed), catch basin (for washing hair in bed), chair (for washing hair in sink), large garbage bag or plastic sheet (for washing hair in sink), comb and brush, hair dryer

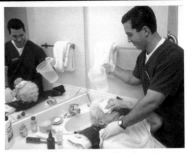

Fig. 4-55. *Make sure the client's head and neck are supported and her eyes covered when washing hair in the sink.*

1. Wash your hands.

2. Explain the procedure to the client, speaking clearly, slowly, and directly. Maintain face-to-face contact whenever possible.

3. Provide privacy for the client. Be sure the room is a comfortable temperature and there are no drafts.

4. Position the client and wet the client's hair.

a. *For washing hair in the sink*, seat the client in a chair covered with plastic. Use a pillow under the plastic to support the head and neck. Have the client lean her head back toward the sink. Give the client a folded washcloth to hold over her forehead or eyes. Wet hair using a plastic cup or a hand-held sink attachment (Fig. 4-55).

b. *For washing hair in the tub*, have the client tilt her head back. Give the client a folded washcloth to hold over her forehead or eyes. Wet hair using a plastic cup or hand-held shower attachment.

c. *For washing hair in the shower*, have the client turn so her back is toward the showerhead. Ask the client to tilt her head backward. Direct the flow of water over the hair to wet it.

d. *For washing hair in bed*, arrange the supplies within reach on a nearby table. Remove all pillows, and place the client in a flat position. If the bed is adjustable, adjust bed to a safe working level, usually waist high. If the bed is movable, lock bed wheels. Place a waterproof pad beneath the client's head and shoulders. Cover the client with the cotton blanket, and fold back the top sheet and regular blankets. Place the trough under the client's head and connect trough to the catch basin. Using the pitcher, pour enough water on the client's hair to make it thoroughly wet.

5. Apply a small amount of shampoo to your hands and rub them together. Using both hands, massage the shampoo to a lather in the client's hair. With your fingertips, massage

the scalp in a circular motion, from front to back (Fig. 4-56). Do not scratch the scalp.

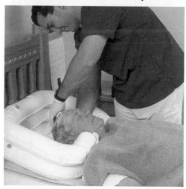

Fig. 4-56. Use your fingertips to work shampoo into a lather. Be gentle so that you do not scratch the scalp.

6. Rinse the hair in the same way you wet it. Rinse until water runs clear. Repeat the shampoo, rinse again, and use conditioner if the client wants it. Be sure to rinse the hair thoroughly to prevent the client's scalp from getting dry and itchy.

7. Wrap the client's hair in a towel. If shampooing at the sink, return the client to an upright position. If shampooing in the bath or shower, assist the client from the tub or shower. If shampooing in bed, remove the trough. Using the washcloth or a face towel, wipe water from the head and neck.

8. Remove the hair towel and gently rub scalp and hair with the towel. Comb or brush hair (see next procedure).

9. Dry hair with a hair dryer on the low setting. Style hair as the client prefers.

10. Wash and store equipment. Put soiled towels and washcloth in the hamper or laundry basket. If you raised an adjustable bed, return it to its lowest position.

11. Wash your hands.

12. Document the procedure and your observations. How did the client tolerate having her hair washed? Was the client able to help? Have the client's abilities changed since the last time her hair was washed?

Handle your clients' hair very carefully. Because hair thins as people age, pieces of hair can be pulled out of the head while combing or brushing it. Be gentle when combing or brushing hair.

Combing or brushing hair

Equipment: comb, brush, towel, mirror, hair care items requested by client

Use hair care products that the client prefers for his or her type of hair.

1. Wash your hands.

2. Explain the procedure to the client, speaking clearly, slowly, and directly. Maintain face-to-face contact whenever possible.

3. Provide privacy for the client.

4. If the client is confined to bed, raise the head of the bed, use a backrest, or use pillows to raise the client's head and shoul-

ders. If the bed is adjustable, adjust bed to a safe working level, usually waist high. If the bed is movable, lock bed wheels. If the client is ambulatory, provide a chair.

5. Place the towel under the client's head or around the shoulders.

6. Remove any hairpins, hair ties, and clips.

7. If the hair is tangled, work on the tangles first. Remove tangles by dividing hair into small sections. Hold the lock of hair just above the tangle so you do not pull at the scalp, and gently comb or brush through the tangle (Fig. 4-57). Gently comb out from ends of hair to scalp. If client agrees, you can use a small amount of detangler or leave-in conditioner on the tangle.

8. After tangles are removed, brush two-inch sections of hair at a time. Brush from roots to ends.

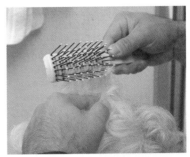

Fig. 4-57. Gently brush hair from roots to ends.

9. Each client may prefer a different hairstyle. Style hair in the way the client prefers. Avoid childish hairstyles. Offer a mirror to the client.

10. Remove the towel and shake excess hair in the wastebasket. Place the soiled towel in the hamper. Store supplies. Clean hair from brush/comb. If you raised an adjustable bed, return it to its lowest position.

11. Wash your hands.

12. Document the procedure and any observations.

Nail care should be provided if it has been assigned or if nails are dirty or have jagged edges. Never cut a client's toenails. In some clients, poor circulation can lead to infection if skin is accidentally cut while caring for nails. In a diabetic client, such an infection can lead to a severe wound or even amputation. If you are directed to provide nail care, know exactly what care you need to provide.

Providing fingernail care

Equipment: orangewood stick, emery board, small basin or bowl, bath thermometer (if available), washcloth, lotion, 2 towels, soap, gloves

1. Wash your hands.

2. Explain the procedure to the client, speaking clearly, slowly, and directly. Maintain face-to-face contact whenever possible.

3. Provide privacy for the client.

4. If the bed is adjustable, adjust bed to a safe working level, usually waist high. If the bed is movable, lock bed wheels.

5. If necessary, remove nail polish with a cotton ball soaked with nail polish remover.

6. Fill the basin halfway with warm water. Test water temperature with the bath thermometer or with your wrist to ensure it is safe. Water temperature should be 105°F. Have the client check the water temperature on his or her wrist. Adjust if necessary. Place basin at a comfortable level for the client.

7. Put on gloves.

8. Soak the client's hands and nails in the basin of water. Soak all 10 fingertips for at least five minutes.

9. Remove hands from water. Wash hands with soapy washcloth. Rinse. Pat hands dry with towel, including between fingers. Remove the hand basin.

10. Place client's hands on the towel. Clean under each fingernail with orangewood stick (Fig. 4-58).

11. Wipe orangewood stick on towel after each nail. Wash client's hands again. Dry them thoroughly, especially between fingers.

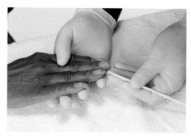

Fig. 4-58. Be gentle when removing dirt from under the nails with an orangewood stick.

12. Shape nails with file or emery board. File in a curve. Finish with nails smooth and free of rough edges.

13. Apply lotion from fingertips to wrists.

14. Discard the water and clean the basin. Dispose of the towels in the laundry hamper and store supplies. If you raised an adjustable bed, return it to its lowest position. Discard gloves.

15. Wash your hands.

16. Document procedure and any observations.

Providing foot care

Equipment: basin, bath mat, 2 bath towels, washcloth, lotion, soap, bath thermometer, gloves, clean socks

1. Wash your hands.

2. Explain the procedure to the client, speaking clearly, slowly, and directly. Maintain face-to-face contact whenever possible.

3. Provide privacy for the client.

4. If client is in bed, and the bed is adjustable, adjust bed to a safe working level, usually waist high. If the bed is movable, lock bed wheels.

5. Fill the basin halfway with warm water. Test water temperature with the bath thermometer or with your wrist to ensure it is safe. Water temperature should be 105°F. Have the client check the water temperature on his or her wrist. Adjust if necessary.

6. Place basin on a bath mat or bath towel on the floor (if the client is sitting in a chair) or on a towel at the foot of the bed (if the client is in bed). Make sure basin is in a comfortable position for client.

7. Put on gloves.

8. Remove client's socks. Completely submerge the client's feet in water. Soak the feet for five to ten minutes. Add warm water to the basin as necessary.

9. Put soap on wet washcloth. Remove one foot from water. Wash entire foot, including between the toes and around nail beds (Fig. 4-59).

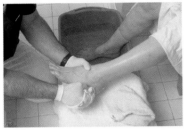

Fig. 4-59. *Soak the client's feet first before washing the entire foot, including the nail beds.*

10. Rinse entire foot, including between the toes.

11. Thoroughly dry entire foot, including between the toes.

12. Repeat steps 9-11 for other foot.

13. Put lotion in one hand and warm the lotion by rubbing hands together.

14. Massage lotion into entire foot (top and bottom), except between toes. Remove excess (if any) with a towel.

15. Help client to replace socks.

16. Discard the water and clean the basin. Dispose of the towels in the laundry hamper and store supplies. If you raised an adjustable bed, return it to its lowest position. Remove and discard gloves.

17. Wash your hands.

18. Document procedure and any observations. Was there any redness, whiteness, or broken or discolored skin? Were there any differences in temperature?

Make sure the client wants you to shave him or help him shave before you begin. Respect personal preferences for shaving. Always wear gloves when shaving a client.

Shaving a client

Equipment: razor, basin filled halfway with warm water (if using a safety or disposable razor), shaving cream or soap (if using a safety or disposable razor), 2 towels, washcloth, mirror, after-shave lotion, gloves

1. Wash your hands.

2. Explain the procedure to the client, speaking clearly, slowly, and directly. Maintain face-to-face contact whenever possible.

3. Provide privacy for the client.

4. Place the equipment on a table within reach of the client if he will shave himself. If the client is confined to bed, raise the head of the bed, use a backrest, or use pillows to raise the client's head and shoulders. If the bed is adjustable, adjust bed to a safe working level, usually waist high. If the bed is movable, lock bed wheels. If the client wears dentures, be sure they are in place. Place the towel across the client's chest, under the client's chin.

5. Put on gloves.

Shaving using a safety or disposable razor:

6. If using a safety or disposable razor, use a blade that is sharp. A dull blade is hard on the skin. Soften the beard with a warm, wet washcloth on the face before shaving. Lather the face with shaving cream or soap and warm water. Warm water and lather make shaving more comfortable.

7. Hold skin taut. Shave in the direction of hair growth. Shave beard in downward strokes on face and upward strokes on neck (Fig. 4-60). Rinse the blade often in warm water to keep it clean and wet.

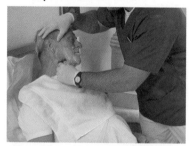

Fig. 4-60. Holding the skin taut, shave in downward strokes on face and upward strokes on neck.

8. When you have finished, wash, rinse, and dry the client's face with a warm, wet washcloth or let him use the washcloth himself. Offer a mirror to the client.

Shaving using an electric razor:

6. Use a small brush to clean razor. Do not use an electric razor near any water source, when oxygen is in use, or if client has a pacemaker.

7. Turn on the razor and hold skin taut. Shave with smooth, even movements (Fig. 4-61). Shave beard with back and forth motion in direction of beard growth with foil shaver. Shave beard in circular motion with three-head shaver. Shave the chin and under the chin.

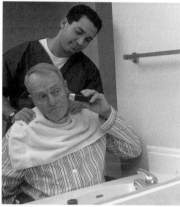

Fig. 4-61. Shave with smooth, even movements.

8. Offer a mirror to the client.

Final steps:

9. Apply after-shave lotion as the client wishes.

10. Remove the towel. Put the towel and washcloth in the hamper or laundry basket. If you raised an adjustable bed, return it to its lowest position.

11. Clean the equipment and store it. For safety razor, rinse the razor. For disposable razor, dispose of it in a sharps container if available. For electric razor, clean head of razor. Remove whiskers from razor. Recap shaving head and return razor to case.

12. Remove and discard gloves.

13. Wash your hands.

14. Document the procedure and any observations.

Guidelines: Helping a Client Dress and Undress

G   Ask about and follow the client's preferences.

G   Allow the client to choose clothing for the day. However, check to see if it is clean, appropriate for the weather, and in good condition.

G   Encourage the client to dress in regular clothes rather than night-clothes.

G   The client should do as much to dress or undress himself as possible.

G   Provide privacy.

G   Roll or fold socks or stockings so they can be slipped over toes and foot, then unrolled into place.

G   For a female client, make sure bra cups fit over the breasts. Front-fastening bras are easier for clients to manage by themselves.

G   If a client has a weakened side due to a stroke or injury, that side is called the "affected" or "involved" side. It will be weaker. Use the terms "affected" or "involved" to refer to the weaker side. Never refer to the weaker side as the "bad" side or talk about the "bad" leg or arm.

G   Place the weak arm or leg through the garment first, then the strong arm. When undressing, do the opposite.

G   Assistive devices for dressing are available. They help maintain independence. Use them as directed.

Oral Care

Oral care, or care of the mouth, teeth, and gums, is performed at least twice each day. Oral care should be done after breakfast and after the last meal or snack of the day. It may also be done before a client eats. Oral care includes brushing teeth, gums, and tongue; flossing teeth; and caring for dentures. When giving oral care, wear gloves. Follow Standard Precautions. When you assist with oral care, observe the client's mouth.

Observing and Reporting: Oral Care

O/R   Irritation

O/R   Infection

O/R   Raised areas

O/R   Coated or swollen tongue

°/R Ulcers, such as canker sores or small, painful, white sores

°/R Flaky, white spots

°/R Dry, cracked, bleeding, or chapped lips

°/R Loose, chipped, broken, or decayed teeth

°/R Swollen, irritated, bleeding, or whitish gums

°/R Breath that smells bad or fruity

°/R Client reports of mouth pain

Providing oral care

Equipment: toothbrush, toothpaste, emesis basin, glass of water, bath towel, gloves

1. Wash your hands.

2. Explain the procedure to the client, speaking clearly, slowly, and directly. Maintain face-to-face contact whenever possible.

3. Provide privacy for the client.

4. If your client is in bed, raise the head of the bed, use a backrest, or use pillows to have him in an upright sitting position. If the bed is adjustable, adjust bed to a safe working level, usually waist high. If the bed is movable, lock bed wheels.

5. Put on gloves.

6. Place a towel across the client's chest.

7. Remove any dental bridgework or ask your client to do so.

8. Wet toothbrush and put a small amount of toothpaste on it.

9. Clean entire mouth (including tongue and all surfaces of the teeth). Use gentle strokes. First brush upper teeth, then lower teeth. Use short strokes. Brush back and forth.

10. Give the client water to rinse the mouth. Place emesis basin under the client's chin, with the inward curve under the cli-ent's bottom lip. Have client spit water into emesis basin (Fig. 4-62). Wipe the client's mouth and remove towel.

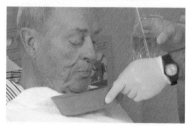

Fig. 4-62. Rinsing and spitting removes food particles and toothpaste.

11. Replace any dental bridgework. Apply moisturizer to the lips if the client desires.

12. Put the soiled towels in the laundry hamper. Dispose of the water in the basin by pouring it into the toilet. Clean the basin and put away supplies. If you raised an adjustable bed, return it to its lowest position. Remove and discard gloves.

13. Wash your hands.

14. Document the procedure and any observations. Did you observe any mouth ulcers or other broken skin? What was the condition of the mucous membrane? Did the client's breath smell unusual?

Although unconscious clients cannot eat, breathing through the mouth causes saliva to dry in the mouth. Good oral care needs to be performed more frequently to keep the mouth clean and moist. Swabs with a mixture of lemon juice and glycerine are sometimes used to soothe the gums. However, these may further dry the gums if used too often. Follow the care plan regarding the use of swabs.

With unconscious clients, use as little liquid as possible when performing oral care. Because the person's swallowing reflex is weak, he or she is at risk for aspiration. **Aspiration** is the inhalation of food, fluid, or foreign material into the lungs. Aspiration can cause pneumonia or death. Turning unconscious clients on their sides before giving oral care can also help prevent aspiration.

Providing oral care for the unconscious client

Equipment: sponge swabs, padded tongue blade, emesis basin or small bowl, towel, glass of cool water, cleaning solution (as ordered in the care plan), lip moisturizer, gloves

1. Wash your hands.

2. Explain the procedure to the client, speaking clearly, slowly, and directly. Maintain face-to-face contact whenever possible. Even clients who are unconscious may be able to hear you. Always speak to them as you would to any client.

3. Provide privacy for the client.

4. If the bed is adjustable, adjust bed to a safe working level, usually waist high. If the bed is movable, lock bed wheels.

5. Put on gloves.

6. Turn your client's head to the side. Place a towel under his cheek and chin. Place emesis basin or bowl next to the cheek and chin for excess fluid.

7. Hold mouth open with the padded tongue blade.

8. Dip the sponge swab in the cleaning solution. Squeeze excess solution to prevent aspi-

ration. Wipe teeth, gums, tongue, and inside surfaces of the mouth. Remove debris with the swab. Change swab often. Repeat this step until the mouth is clean (Fig. 4-63).

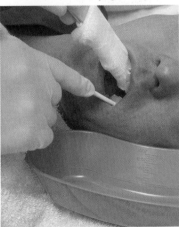

Fig. 4-63. Wipe all inside surfaces of the mouth to clean the mouth, stimulate the gums, and remove mucus.

9. Rinse with clean swab dipped in water. Squeeze swab first to remove excess water.

10. Remove the towel and basin. Pat lips or face dry if needed. Apply lip moisturizer.

11. Place the towel in the laundry hamper. Clean the basin and put away supplies. If you raised an adjustable bed, return it to its lowest position. Remove and discard gloves.

12. Wash your hands.

13. Document the procedure and your observations. Did you observe any mouth ulcers or other broken skin? What was the condition of the mucous membrane? Did the client's breath smell unusual?

Flossing the teeth removes plaque and tartar buildup around the gum line and between the teeth. Teeth may be flossed immediately after or before they are brushed. Follow the client's preference.

Flossing teeth

Equipment: dental floss, glass of water, emesis basin, face towel, gloves

1. Wash your hands.

2. Explain the procedure to the client, speaking clearly, slowly, and directly. Maintain face-to-face contact whenever possible.

3. Provide privacy for the client.

4. If your client is in bed, raise the head of the bed, use a backrest, or use pillows to have him in an upright sitting position. If the bed is adjustable, adjust bed to a safe working level, usually waist high. If the bed is movable, lock bed wheels.

5. Put on gloves.

6. Wrap the ends of the floss securely around each of your index fingers (Fig. 4-64).

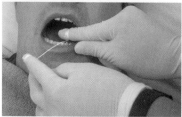

Fig. 4-64. *Before beginning, wrap floss securely around each index finger.*

7. Starting with the back teeth, place the floss between teeth and move it down the surface of the tooth using a gentle sawing motion. Continue to the gum line. At the gum line, curve the floss into a letter C. Slip it gently into the space between the gum and tooth, then go back up, scraping that side of the tooth. Repeat this on the side of the other tooth.

8. After every two teeth, unwind floss from your fingers and move it so you are using a clean area. Floss all teeth.

9. Occasionally offer water so that the client can rinse debris from the mouth into the basin.

10. Offer the client a face towel when done flossing all teeth.

11. Discard floss. Pour water from the basin into the toilet. Clean and store the basin. Put the soiled face towel in the laundry hamper. If you raised an adjustable bed, return it to its lowest position. Remove and discard gloves.

12. Wash your hands.

13. Document procedure and observations.

Dentures are artificial teeth. They are expensive, so take good care of them. Handle dentures carefully to avoid breaking or chipping them. If a client's dentures break, he or she cannot eat. When cleaning dentures, wear gloves. Notify your supervisor if a client's dentures do not fit properly, are chipped, or are missing. Ask the client how you can assist with denture care. Each person has his own preference about when and how it should be done.

Cleaning and storing dentures

Equipment: denture brush or soft toothbrush, denture cleaner or tablet, denture cup, 2 towels, gauze squares, gloves

1. Wash your hands.

2. Explain the procedure to the client, speaking clearly, slowly, and directly. Maintain face-to-face contact whenever possible.

3. Provide privacy for the client.

4. Put on gloves.

5. Line the sink or a basin with one or two face towels and partially fill with water. The towel and water will prevent the dentures from breaking if they slip from your hands and fall into the sink.

6. Ask the client to remove the dentures and place them in the denture cup. If the client is unable to remove them, do it yourself. Remove the lower denture first. The lower denture is easier to remove because it floats on the gum line of the lower jaw. Grasp the lower denture with a gauze square (for a good grip) and remove it. Place it in a denture cup filled with cool water.

7. The upper denture is sealed by suction. Firmly grasp the upper denture with a gauze square and give a slight downward pull to break the suction. Turn it at an angle to take it out of the mouth.

8. Take the denture cup to the sink or basin. Rinse dentures in cool running water before brushing them. Do not use hot water, or dentures may warp.

9. Apply toothpaste or cleanser to toothbrush.

10. Brush dentures on all surfaces (Fig. 4-65).

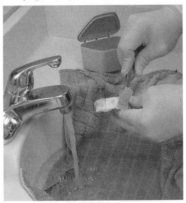

Fig. 4-65. Brush dentures on all surfaces to properly clean them.

11. Rinse all surfaces of dentures under cool running water. Do not use hot water.

12. Rinse denture cup before placing clean dentures in the cup.

13. Your client may prefer to clean the dentures with a soaking solution. Read the directions on the bottle and prepare the solution. Soak the dentures for the amount of time indicated. Rinse and place in denture cup.

14. Store dentures in solution or cool water to prevent them from warping. Place lid on cup. To avoid accidentally throwing dentures away, always store them in a labeled denture cup when the client is not wearing them. Some clients will want to wear dentures all of the time.

They will only remove them for cleaning.

15. Drain sink. Put towels in laundry hamper. Rinse and store toothbrush and other supplies. Remove and discard gloves.

16. Wash your hands.

17. Document procedure and any observations.

Reinserting dentures

Equipment: denture cup with dentures, denture cream or adhesive, face towel, gloves

Ask if the client needs your assistance in inserting dentures.

1. Wash your hands.

2. Explain the procedure to the client, speaking clearly, slowly, and directly. Maintain face-to-face contact whenever possible.

3. Provide privacy for the client.

4. Position client as you would for brushing teeth (help him to as upright a position as possible).

5. Put on gloves.

6. Apply denture cream or adhesive to the dentures if needed.

7. Ask client to open his or her mouth. Insert the upper denture into the mouth by turning it at an angle. Straighten it and press it onto the upper gum line firmly and evenly (Fig. 4-66).

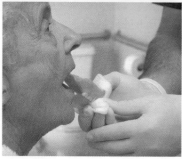

Fig. 4-66. Press upper denture onto the upper gum line firmly and evenly.

8. Insert the lower denture onto the gum line of the lower jaw and press firmly.

9. Offer the client the face towel.

10. Rinse and store the denture cup. Remove and discard gloves.

11. Wash your hands.

12. Document the procedure and any observations.

Toileting

Clients who are unable to get out of bed to go to the bathroom may be given a bedpan, a fracture pan, or a urinal. A fracture pan is a bedpan that is flatter than a regular bedpan. It is used for clients who cannot assist with raising their hips onto a regular bedpan. Women will generally use a bedpan for urination and bowel movements. Men will generally use a urinal for urination and a bedpan for a bowel movement.

Some clients are able to get out of bed, but may still need help walking to the bathroom and using the toilet. Others who are able to get out of bed but cannot walk to the bathroom may use a portable commode. A portable commode is a chair with a toilet seat and a removable container underneath. Toilets can be fitted with raised seats to make it easier for clients to get up and down. Hand rails can also be installed next to the toilet. Observe and report if these assistive devices are needed but not present. When clients need assistance to get to the bathroom or use the commode, offer to help often. This can avoid accidents and embarrassment.

Remember that wastes such as urine and feces can carry infection. Always dispose of wastes in the toilet. Be careful not to spill or splash. Wear gloves when handling bedpans, urinals, or basins that contain wastes, including dirty bath water. Wash these containers thoroughly. After washing these containers, remove your gloves and wash your hands. Put on a new pair of gloves if you are not finished with client care.

Washcloths used to wash perineal areas must be washed in hot water. Handle such laundry carefully, and wear gloves. Washing it separately is safest. Disposable washcloths may or may not be flushable. Read the package to be sure. If they are not flushable, dispose of them in a waste container lined with a plastic bag. Remove and replace the plastic bag frequently to prevent odors.

Assisting client with use of a bedpan

Equipment: bedpan, bedpan cover (newspaper or washable cloth), protective pad or sheet, bath blanket, toilet paper, disposable washcloths or wipes, soap, towel, plastic bag, 2 pairs of gloves

1. **Wash your hands.**

2. **Explain the procedure to the client, speaking clearly, slowly, and directly. Maintain face-to-face contact whenever possible.**

3. **Provide privacy for the client by closing doors and shades and using a covering blanket.**

4. **If the bed is adjustable, adjust bed to a safe working level, usually waist high. Before placing bedpan, lower the head of the bed. If the bed is movable, lock bed wheels.**

5. **Put on gloves.**

6. **Warm outside of the bedpan with warm water in the bathroom and cover it when you bring it to the client. Dust the top of the bedpan with powder to prevent it from sticking to the client's skin. Do not use talcum powder if the client has open sores on the buttocks or genitals. Do not use powder if a stool or urine sample is needed. If a stool or urine sample is not needed, place a few sheets of toilet paper in the bedpan to make cleanup easier.**

7. **Cover the client with the bath blanket and ask him to hold it while you pull down the top covers underneath it. Do not expose more of client than you have to.**

8. Place a protective pad under the client's buttocks and hips. To do this, have the client roll toward you. If the client cannot do this, you must turn the client toward you. Be sure the client cannot roll off the bed. Move to the empty side of the bed. Place the protective pad on the area where the client will lie on his back. The side of the protective pad nearest the client should be fanfolded (folded several times into pleats) (Fig. 4-67).

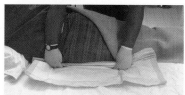

Fig. 4-67. Fanfold the bed protector near the client's back.

Ask the client to roll onto his back, or roll him as you did before. Unfold the rest of the protective pad so it completely covers the area under and around the client's hips (Fig. 4-68).

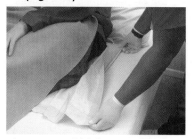

Fig. 4-68. Unfold the rest of the bed protector so it completely covers area under and around the client's hips.

9. Ask the client to remove undergarments, or help him do so.

10. Place the bedpan near his hips in the correct position.

Standard bedpan should be positioned with the wider end aligned with the client's buttocks. Fracture pan should be positioned with handle toward foot of the bed.

11. If client is able, ask him to raise hips by pushing with feet and hands at the count of three (Fig. 4-69). Slide the bedpan under his hips.

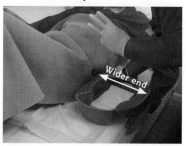

Fig. 4-69. On the count of three, slide the bedpan under the client's hips. The wider end of bedpan should be aligned with the client's buttocks.

If the client cannot do this himself, place your arm under the small of his back. Tell him to push with his heels and hands on your signal as you raise his hips (Fig. 4-70).

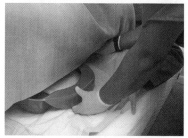

Fig. 4-70. If a client cannot raise his hips, you can raise his hips while he pushes with his heels and hands.

If a client cannot help you in any way, keep the bed flat and roll the client onto the far side. Slip the bedpan under the hips and gently roll the client back onto the bedpan. Keep the bedpan centered underneath.

12. Remove and discard gloves. Wash your hands.

13. Raise the head of the bed. Prop the client into a semi-sitting position using pillows.

14. Make sure the bath blanket is still covering the client. Place toilet paper, washcloths or wipes, and a bell or other way to call you within client's reach. Ask client to clean his hands with the hand wipe when finished, if he is able.

15. Tell the client you will return when called. Leave the room.

16. When called by the client, return and put on clean gloves.

17. Lower the head of the bed. Make sure client is still covered.

18. Remove bedpan carefully and cover bedpan.

19. Provide perineal care if help is needed. For female clients, wipe from the front to the back.

Dry the perineal area with a towel. Help the client put on undergarment. Place the towel in a hamper or bag, and discard disposable supplies.

20. Take bedpan to the bathroom. Empty the bedpan carefully into the toilet unless a specimen is needed. Note color, odor, and consistency of contents before flushing. If you notice anything unusual about the stool or urine (for example, the presence of blood), do not discard it. You will need to notify your supervisor.

21. Using a paper towel, turn the faucet on. Rinse the bedpan with cold water first and empty it into the toilet. Then clean the bedpan with hot, soapy water and store.

22. Remove and discard gloves.

23. Wash your hands.

24. If you raised an adjustable bed, return it to its lowest position.

25. Document the time of the elimination, the contents, and any observations.

Assisting a male client with a urinal

Equipment: urinal, protective pad or sheet, washcloths or wipes, soap, 2 pairs of gloves

1. Wash your hands.

2. Explain the procedure to the client, speaking clearly, slowly, and directly. Maintain face-to-face contact whenever possible.

3. Provide privacy for the client by closing doors and shades and using a covering blanket.

4. If the bed is adjustable, adjust bed to a safe working level,

usually waist high. If the bed is movable, lock bed wheels.

5. Put on gloves.

6. Place a protective pad under the client's buttocks and hips, as in earlier procedure.

7. Hand the urinal to the client. If the client is not able to help himself, place the urinal between his legs and position the penis inside the urinal (Fig. 4-71). Replace covers.

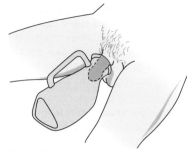

Fig. 4-71. Position the penis inside the urinal if the client cannot do it himself.

8. Remove and discard gloves. Wash your hands.

9. Place wipes within client's reach. Ask the client to clean his hands with the hand wipe when finished, if he is able. Give the client a bell or another way to call you. Ask client to signal when done. Leave the room.

10. When called by the client, return and put on clean gloves.

11. Remove the urinal, or have client hand it to you. Empty contents into toilet unless a specimen is needed or the client's urine is being measured for intake/output monitoring. Note color, odor, and qualities (for example, cloudiness) of contents before flushing.

12. Using a paper towel, turn the faucet on. Rinse the urinal with cold water and empty it into the toilet. Store it.

13. Remove and discard gloves. Wash your hands.

14. If you raised an adjustable bed, return it to its lowest position.

15. Document the time, the amount of urine (if monitoring intake and output), and any other observations.

Assisting a client to use a portable commode or toilet

Equipment: portable commode with basin (Fig. 4-72), toilet paper, disposable washcloths or wipes, towel, gloves

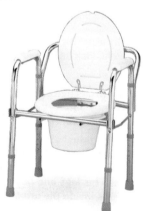

Fig. 4-72. One type of portable commode. (PHOTO COURTESY OF NOVA ORTHO MED, INC.)

1. Wash your hands.

2. Explain the procedure to the client, speaking clearly, slowly, and directly. Maintain face-to-face contact whenever possible.

3. Provide privacy for the client by closing doors and shades and using a covering blanket.

4. Help client out of bed and to the portable commode or bathroom. Make sure client is wearing non-skid shoes and that the laces are tied.

5. If needed, help client remove clothing and sit comfortably on toilet seat. Put toilet tissue and washcloths or wipes within reach. Ask client to clean his hands with the hand wipes when finished, if he is able.

6. Provide privacy. Give the client a bell or another way to call you. Leave the room and close the door, but do not lock it. Do not go too far away in case you are needed soon.

7. When called by the client, return and put on gloves. Give perineal care if help is needed. Wipe female residents from front to back. Dry the perineal area with a towel. Help the resident put on undergarment. Place the towel in a hamper or bag. Discard disposable supplies.

8. Help the client up and back to bed.

9. When using a portable commode, remove waste container and empty it into the toilet unless a specimen is needed or the client's urine is being measured for intake/output monitoring. Note color, odor, and consistency of contents before flushing.

10. Clean the container as you would a bedpan, rinsing first with cold water and then washing with hot water and cleanser.

11. Remove and discard gloves. Wash your hands.

12. If you raised an adjustable bed, return it to its lowest position.

13. Document the procedure and any observations.

Vital Signs

Home health aides monitor, document, and report clients' vital signs. Vital signs are important. They show how well the vital organs of the body, such as the heart and lungs, are working. They consist of the following:

- Measuring the body temperature
- Counting the pulse 60-100
- Counting the rate of respirations 12-20
- Measuring the blood pressure
- Observing and reporting the level of pain

Watching for changes in vital signs is very important. Changes can indicate that a client's condition is worsening. Always notify your supervisor if:

- The client has a fever (temperature is above average for the client or outside the normal range)
- The client has a respiratory or pulse rate that is too rapid or too slow
- The client's blood pressure changes
- The client's pain is worse or is not relieved by pain management

Normal Ranges for Vital Signs

Temperature	Fahrenheit	Celsius
Oral	97.6°–99.6°	36.5°–37.5°
Rectal	98.6°–100.6°	37.0°–38.1°
Axillary	96.6°–98.6°	36.0°–37.0°

Pulse: 60–100 beats per minute
Respirations: 12–20 respirations per minute

Blood Pressure
Normal: Systolic 100–139 Diastolic 60–89
High: 140/90 or above
Low: Below 100/60

Temperature

Body temperature is normally very close to 98.6°F (Fahrenheit) or 37°C (Celsius). Body temperature is a balance between the heat created by our bodies and the heat lost to the environment. Many factors affect temperature: age, illness, stress, environment, exercise, and the circadian rhythm can all cause changes in body temperature. The circadian rhythm is the 24-hour day-night cycle. Increases in body temperature may indicate an infection or disease. There are four sites for taking body temperature:

1. The mouth (oral)

2. The rectum (rectal)

3. The armpit (axillary)

4. The ear (tympanic)

The different sites require different thermometers. Temperatures are most often taken orally. Remember that there is a range of normal temperatures. Some people's temperatures normally run low. Others in completely good health will run slightly higher temperatures. Normal temperature readings also vary according to the method used to take the temperature. A rectal temperature is considered to be the most accurate. Types of thermometers are:

• Mercury-free glass

• Mercury glass (glass bulb)

• Battery-powered, digital, or electronic

• Disposable

- Tympanic
- Temporal artery

Using mercury glass or glass bulb thermometers to take oral or rectal temperatures used to be common. However, because mercury is a dangerous, toxic substance, many facilities now do not use products containing mercury. In fact, many states have passed laws to ban the sale of mercury thermometers.

Today, mercury-free glass thermometers are more common (Fig. 4-73). They can be used to take an oral or rectal temperature, and they are considered much safer. Mercury-free thermometers can usually be purchased at your local pharmacy.

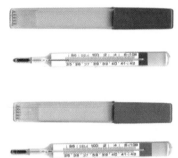

Fig. 4-73. A *mercury-free oral thermometer and a mercury-free rectal thermometer. Thermometers are usually color-coded to show which is an oral and which is a rectal thermometer. Oral thermometers are usually green or blue; rectal thermometers are usually red.* (PHOTOS PROVIDED BY RG MEDICAL DIAGNOSTICS OF SOUTHFIELD, MI.)

Measuring and recording oral temperature

Do not take an oral temperature on a client who has smoked, had food or fluids, chewed gum, or exercised in the last 10–20 minutes.

Equipment: clean mercury-free, digital, or electronic thermometer, gloves, disposable plastic sheath/cover for thermometer, tissues, pen and paper

1. **Wash your hands.**
2. **Explain the procedure to the client, speaking clearly, slowly, and directly. Maintain face-to-face contact whenever possible.**
3. **Provide privacy for the client.**
4. **Put on gloves.**
5. *Mercury-free thermometer:* **Hold the thermometer by the stem. Before inserting the thermometer in the client's mouth, shake thermometer down to below the lowest number (at** least below 96°F or 35°C). **To shake the thermometer down, hold it at the side opposite the bulb with the thumb and two fingers. With a snapping motion of the wrist, shake the thermometer (Fig. 4-74). Stand away from furniture and walls while doing so.**

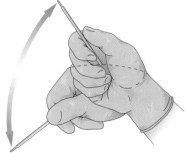

Fig. 4-74. Shake thermometer down to below the lowest number before inserting in a client's mouth.

Digital thermometer: Put on the disposable sheath. Turn on thermometer and wait until "ready" sign appears.

Electronic thermometer: Remove the probe from base unit. Put on probe cover.

6. *Mercury-free thermometer*: Put on disposable sheath, if available. Insert bulb end of the thermometer into client's mouth, under tongue and to one side (Fig. 4-75).

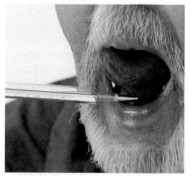

Fig. 4-75. Insert thermometer under the client's tongue and to one side.

Digital thermometer: Insert the end of digital thermometer into client's mouth, under tongue and to one side.

Electronic thermometer: Insert the end of electronic thermometer into client's mouth, under tongue and to one side.

7. *Mercury-free thermometer*: Tell the client to hold the thermometer in mouth with lips closed. Assist as necessary. Client should breathe through his nose. Ask the client not to bite down or to talk. Leave the thermometer in place for at least three minutes.

Digital thermometer: Leave in place until thermometer blinks or beeps.

Electronic thermometer: Leave in place until you hear a tone or see a flashing or steady light.

8. *Mercury-free thermometer*: Remove the thermometer. Wipe with a tissue from stem to bulb or remove sheath. Dispose of the tissue or sheath. Hold the thermometer at eye level. Rotate until line appears, rolling the thermometer between your thumb and forefinger. Read the temperature. Remember the temperature reading.

Digital thermometer: Remove the thermometer. Read temperature on display screen. Remember the temperature reading.

Electronic thermometer: Read the temperature on the display screen. Remember the temperature reading. Remove the probe from the mouth.

9. *Mercury-free thermometer*: Rinse the thermometer in lukewarm water and dry. Return it to a plastic case or container.

Digital thermometer: Using a tissue, remove and dispose of sheath. Replace the thermometer in case.

Electronic thermometer: Press the eject button to discard the cover. Return the probe to the holder.

10. Remove and discard gloves.

11. Wash your hands.

12. Immediately record the temperature, date, time, and method used (oral).

Always explain what you will do before taking a rectal temperature. Advise the client to hold still. Reassure him that the procedure will only take a few minutes. Keep your hand on the thermometer the entire time you are taking the temperature.

Measuring and recording a rectal temperature

Equipment: clean rectal mercury-free or digital thermometer, lubricant, gloves, tissue, disposable sheath/cover, pen and paper

1. Wash your hands.

2. Explain the procedure to the client, speaking clearly, slowly, and directly. Maintain face-to-face contact whenever possible.

3. Provide privacy for the client.

4. Assist the client to a left-lying (Sims') position. An infant can be placed on his back or stomach for measuring rectal temperature.

5. Fold back the linens to expose only the rectal area.

6. Put on gloves.

7. *Mercury-free thermometer:* Hold thermometer by stem. Shake the thermometer down to below the lowest number.

   Digital thermometer: Put on the disposable sheath. Turn on thermometer and wait until "ready" sign appears.

8. Apply a small amount of lubricant to tip of bulb or probe cover.

9. Separate the buttocks. Gently insert thermometer into rectum one inch (1/2 inch for a child). Stop if you meet resistance. Do not force the thermometer in the rectum (Fig. 4-76).

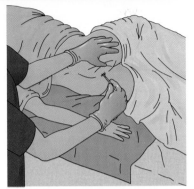

Fig. 4-76. Gently insert a rectal thermometer one inch into the rectum. Do not force it into the rectum.

10. Replace the sheet over buttocks while holding on to the thermometer. Hold on to the thermometer at all times.

11. *Mercury-free thermometer:* Hold thermometer in place for at least three minutes.

    Digital thermometer: Hold thermometer in place until thermometer blinks or beeps.

12. Gently remove the thermometer. Wipe with tissue from stem to bulb or remove sheath.

    Dispose of tissue or sheath.

13. Read the thermometer at eye level as you would for an oral temperature. Remember the temperature reading.

14. *Mercury-free thermometer:* Rinse the thermometer in lukewarm water and dry. Return it to plastic case or container.

Digital thermometer: Discard probe cover. Replace the thermometer in case.

15. Remove and discard gloves.

16. Wash your hands.

17. Assist the client to a position of safety and comfort.

18. Immediately record the temperature, date, time, and method used (rectal).

Reassure the client that this procedure is painless. The short tip of the tympanic thermometer will only go into the ear one-quarter to one-half inch. Follow the manufacturer's instructions.

Measuring and recording tympanic temperature

Equipment: tympanic thermometer, gloves, disposable probe sheath/cover, pen and paper

1. Wash your hands.

2. Explain the procedure to the client, speaking clearly, slowly, and directly. Maintain face-to-face contact whenever possible.

3. Provide privacy for the client.

4. Put on gloves.

5. Put a disposable sheath over earpiece of the thermometer.

6. Position the client's head so that the ear is in front of you. Straighten the ear canal by pulling up and back on the outside edge of the ear for an adult (Fig. 4-77). Pull straight back for infants and children. Insert the covered probe into the ear canal and press the button.

7. Hold thermometer in place either for one second or until thermometer beeps (depends on model).

8. Read temperature. Remember the temperature reading.

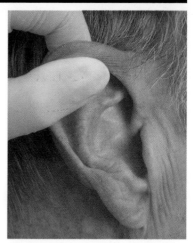

Fig. 4-77. Straighten the ear canal by pulling up and back on the outside edge of the ear.

9. Dispose of sheath. Return the thermometer to storage or to the battery charger if thermometer is rechargeable.

10. Remove and discard gloves.

11. Wash your hands.

12. Immediately record the temperature, date, time, and method used (tympanic).

Measuring and recording axillary temperature

Equipment: clean mercury-free, digital, or electronic thermometer, gloves, tissues, disposable sheath/cover, pen and paper

1. Wash your hands.

2. Explain the procedure to the client, speaking clearly, slowly, and directly. Maintain face-to-face contact whenever possible.

3. Provide privacy for the client.

4. Put on gloves.

5. Remove client's arm from sleeve of gown or top to allow skin contact with the end of thermometer. Wipe axillary area with tissues.

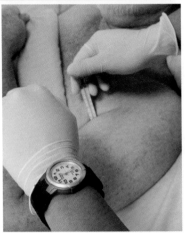

Fig. 4-78. *After inserting the thermometer, fold the client's arm over his chest and hold it in place for eight to ten minutes.*

6. *Mercury-free thermometer*: Hold the thermometer by the stem. Shake the thermometer down to below the lowest number.

   Digital thermometer: Put on the disposable sheath. Turn on thermometer and wait until "ready" sign appears.

   Electronic thermometer: Remove the probe from base unit. Put on probe cover.

7. Position thermometer (bulb end for mercury-free) in center of the armpit. Fold client's arm over his chest.

8. *Mercury-free thermometer*: Hold the thermometer in place, with the arm close against the side, for eight to 10 minutes (Fig. 4-78).

   Digital thermometer: Leave in place until thermometer blinks or beeps.

   Electronic thermometer: Leave in place until you hear a tone or see a flashing or steady light.

9. *Mercury-free thermometer*: Remove the thermometer. Wipe with a tissue from stem to bulb or remove sheath. Dispose of the tissue or sheath. Read the thermometer at eye level as you would for an oral temperature. Remember the temperature reading.

   Digital thermometer: Remove the thermometer. Read temperature on display screen. Remember the temperature reading.

   Electronic thermometer: Read the temperature on the display screen. Remember the temperature reading. Remove the probe.

10. *Mercury-free thermometer*: Rinse the thermometer in lukewarm water and dry. Return it to plastic case or container.

    Digital thermometer: Using a tissue, remove and dispose of sheath. Replace the thermometer in case.

Electronic thermometer: Press the eject button to discard the cover. Return the probe to the holder.

11. Remove and discard gloves.

12. Wash your hands.

13. Immediately record the temperature, date, time, and method used (axillary).

Pulse

The pulse is the number of heartbeats per minute. The beat that you feel at certain pulse points in the body represents the wave of blood moving as a result of the heart pumping. The most common site for checking the pulse is on the inside of the wrist, where the radial artery runs just beneath the skin. This is called the radial pulse. The brachial pulse is the pulse 1–1½ inches upward toward the inside of the elbow. The radial and brachial pulse are involved in taking blood pressure. Blood pressure is explained later in this chapter.

For adults, the normal pulse rate is 60-100 beats per minute. Small children have more rapid pulses, in the range of 100-120 beats per minute. A newborn baby's pulse may be as high as 120-140 beats per minute. Many things can affect the pulse rate, including exercise, fear, anger, anxiety, heat, medications, and pain. An unusually high or low rate does not necessarily indicate disease. However, sometimes the pulse rate can be a signal that serious illness exists. For example, a rapid pulse may result from fever, infection, or heart failure. A slow or weak pulse may indicate dehydration, infection, or shock.

The apical pulse is heard by listening directly over the heart with a stethoscope. A stethoscope is an instrument designed to listen to sounds within the body, such as the heart beating or air moving through the lungs. Measuring apical pulse is often done on infants and small children because their pulse points are harder to find. For adult clients, the apical pulse may be taken when the person has heart disease or takes medication that affects the heart. It may also be taken on clients who have a weak radial pulse or an irregular pulse.

Measuring and recording apical pulse

Equipment: stethoscope, alcohol wipes, watch with second hand, pen and paper

1. Wash your hands.

2. Explain the procedure to the client, speaking clearly, slowly, and directly. Maintain face-to-face contact whenever possible.

3. Provide privacy for the client.

4. Before using the stethoscope, wipe the diaphragm and earpieces of stethoscope with alcohol wipes.

5. Fit the earpieces of the stethoscope in your ears. Place the flat metal diaphragm on the left

side of the chest, just below the nipple (Fig. 4-79). Listen for the heartbeat.

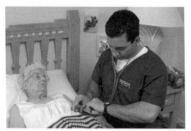

Fig. 4-79. *Count the heartbeats for one full minute to measure the apical pulse.*

6. Use the second hand of your watch. Count the heartbeats for one minute. Each "lubdub" that you hear is counted as one beat. A normal heartbeat is rhythmical. Leave the stethoscope in place to count respirations.

7. Document the pulse rate, date, time, and method used (apical). Note any irregularities in the rhythm.

8. Store stethoscope.

9. Wash your hands.

Respirations

Respiration is the process of breathing air into the lungs, or inspiration, and exhaling air out of the lungs, or expiration. Each respiration consists of an inspiration and an expiration. The chest rises during inspiration and falls during expiration.

The normal respiration rate for adults ranges from 12 to 20 breaths per minute. Infants and children have a faster respiratory rate; infants normally breathe at a rate of 30 to 40 respirations per minute. People may breathe more quickly if they know they are being observed. Because of this, count respirations immediately after taking the pulse. Keep your fingers on the client's wrist or on the stethoscope over the heart. Do not make it obvious that you are observing the client's breathing.

Measuring and recording radial pulse and counting and recording respirations

Equipment: watch with a second hand, pen and paper

1. Wash your hands.

2. Explain the procedure to the client, speaking clearly, slowly, and directly. Maintain face-to-face contact whenever possible.

3. Provide privacy for the client.

4. Place fingertips on the thumb side of client's wrist to locate radial pulse (Fig. 4-80).

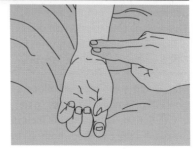

Fig. 4-80. *Measure the radial pulse by placing fingertips on the thumb side of the wrist.*

5. Count the beats for one full minute.

6. Keeping your fingertips on the client's wrist, count respirations for one full minute. Observe for the pattern and character of the client's breathing. Normal breathing is smooth and quiet. If you see signs of difficult breathing, shallow breathing, or noisy breathing, such as wheezing, report it to your supervisor.

7. Document the pulse rate, date, time, and method used (radial). Record the respiratory rate and the pattern or character of breathing. Notify your supervisor if the pulse is less than 60 beats per minute, over 100 beats per minute, or if the rhythm is irregular.

8. Wash your hands.

Blood Pressure

Blood pressure is an important measure of health. Blood pressure is measured in millimeters of mercury (mmHg). The measurement shows how well the heart is working. There are two parts of blood pressure, the **systolic** and **diastolic**.

In the systolic phase, the heart is at work, contracting and pushing the blood from the left ventricle of the heart. The reading shows the pressure on the walls of arteries as blood is pumped through the body. The normal range for systolic blood pressure is 100 to 119 mmHg.

The second measurement reflects the diastolic phase—when the heart relaxes. The diastolic measurement is always lower than the systolic measurement. It shows the pressure in the arteries when the heart is at rest. The normal range for adults is 60 to 79 mmHg.

People with high blood pressure, or hypertension, have elevated systolic and/or diastolic blood pressures. A blood pressure level of 140/90 mmHg or higher is considered high. However, if blood pressure is between 120/80 mmHg and 139/89 mmHg, it is called prehypertension. This means that the person does not have high blood pressure now, but is likely to have it in the future. Report to your supervisor if a client's blood pressure is 140/90 or above.

Many factors can increase blood pressure. These include aging, exercise, physical or emotional stress, pain, medications, and the volume of blood in circulation. This textbook includes one method for measuring blood pressure—the two-step method. In the two-step method, you will get an estimate of the systolic blood pressure before you start. After getting an estimated systolic reading, you will deflate the cuff and begin again. Another method does not require you to get an estimated systolic reading before measuring blood pressure. Follow your agency's policies on which method to use.

Measuring and recording blood pressure (two-step method)

Equipment: sphygmomanometer (blood pressure cuff), stethoscope, alcohol wipes, pen and paper

1. Wash your hands.

2. Explain the procedure to the client, speaking clearly, slowly, and directly. Maintain face-to-face contact whenever possible.

3. Provide privacy for the client.

4. Ask the client to roll up his or her sleeve. Do not measure blood pressure over clothing.

5. Position the client's arm with the palm up. The arm should be level with the heart.

6. With the valve open, squeeze the cuff to make sure it is completely deflated.

7. Place the blood pressure cuff snugly on client's upper arm, with the center of the cuff placed over the brachial artery (1–1½ inches above the elbow toward inside of elbow) (Fig. 4-81).

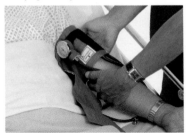

Fig. 4-81. *Place the center of the cuff over the brachial artery.*

8. Locate the radial (wrist) pulse with your fingertips.

9. Close the valve (clockwise) until it stops. Inflate the cuff while watching the gauge.

10. Stop inflating when you can no longer feel the radial pulse. Note the reading. The number is an estimate of the systolic pressure. This estimate helps you not to inflate the cuff too high later in this procedure. Inflating the cuff too high is painful and may damage small blood vessels.

11. Open the valve to deflate cuff completely. An inflated cuff left on client's arm can cause numbness and tingling.

12. Write down the estimated systolic reading.

13. Before using the stethoscope, wipe the diaphragm and earpieces of stethoscope with alcohol wipes.

14. Locate the brachial pulse with fingertips.

15. Place the diaphragm of the stethoscope over the brachial artery.

16. Place the earpieces of the stethoscope in your ears.

17. Close the valve (clockwise) until it stops. Do not tighten it (Fig. 4-82).

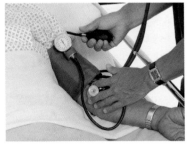

Fig. 4-82. *Close the valve by turning it clockwise until it stops.*

18. Inflate the cuff to 30 mmHg above your estimated systolic pressure.

19. Open the valve slightly with thumb and index finger. Deflate cuff slowly. Releasing the valve slowly allows you to hear beats accurately.

20. Watch the gauge and listen for sound of pulse.

21. Remember the reading at which the first clear pulse sound is heard. This is the systolic pressure.

22. Continue listening for a change or muffling of pulse sound. The point of a change or the point at which the sound disappears is the diastolic pressure. Remember this reading.

23. Open the valve to deflate cuff completely. Remove cuff.

24. Record both systolic and diastolic pressures. Write the numbers like a fraction, with the systolic reading on top and the diastolic reading on the bottom (for example: 120/80). Note which arm was used. Write "RA" for right arm and "LA" for left arm.

25. Wipe diaphragm and earpieces of stethoscope with alcohol. Store equipment.

26. Wash your hands.

Pain

Pain is uncomfortable. It is also a personal experience. This means it is different for each person. It is important to observe and report a client's pain. You play an important role in pain monitoring and prevention. Pain is not a normal part of aging. Treat clients' complaints of pain seriously. If a client complains of pain, ask these questions to get the most accurate information. Report the information to your supervisor immediately.

- Where is the pain?
- When did the pain start?
- Is the pain mild, moderate or severe? To help find out, ask the client to rate the pain on a scale of 0 to 10, with 10 being the worst.
- Ask the client to describe the pain. Make notes if you need to and use the client's words when reporting to your supervisor.
- Ask the client what he or she was doing before the pain started.
- Ask the client how long the pain lasts and how often it occurs.
- Ask the client what makes the pain better and what makes it feel worse.

Measures to reduce pain include the following:
- Report complaints of pain or unrelieved pain promptly to your supervisor.
- Gently position the body in good alignment. Use pillows for support. Assist in frequent changes of position if the client desires it.

- Give back rubs.
- See if the client would like to take a warm bath or shower.
- Help the client to the bathroom or commode or offer the bedpan or urinal.
- Encourage slow, deep breathing.
- Provide a calm and quiet environment. Use soft music to distract the client.
- If a client is taking pain medication, remind him or her when it is time to take it.
- Be patient, caring, gentle, and sympathetic.

Height and Weight

You may be asked to check your clients' weight and height as part of your care. Height is checked less frequently than weight. Weight changes can be signs of illness. They can also affect the medication doses a client needs. For these reasons, you must report any weight loss or gain, no matter how small.

Measuring and recording weight of an ambulatory client

Equipment: bathroom scale or standing scale, pen and paper

1. Wash your hands.

2. Explain the procedure to the client, speaking clearly, slowly, and directly. Maintain face-to-face contact whenever possible.

3. Provide privacy for the client. Some people are sensitive about their weight.

4. If using a bathroom scale, set the scale on a hard surface in a place the client can get to easily.

5. Start with the scale balanced at zero before weighing the client.

6. Help client to step onto the center of the scale. Be sure she is not holding, touching, or leaning against anything. This interferes with weight measure-ment. Do not force someone to let go. If you are unable to obtain a weight, notify your supervisor.

7. Determine the client's weight. *Using a bathroom scale*: read the weight when the dial has stopped moving. *Using a standing scale*: this is done by balancing the scale. Make the balance bar level by moving the small and large weight indicators until the bar balances. Add these two numbers together.

8. Help the client to safely step off scale before recording weight.

9. Document the weight. Report any changes in client's weight to your supervisor.

10. Store the scale if it was moved.

11. Wash your hands.

Measuring and recording height of a client

Some clients will be unable to get out of bed. If so, height can be measured using a tape measure (Fig. 4-83).

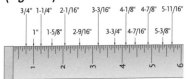

Fig. 4-83. *A tape measure.*

Equipment: tape measure, pencil, pen and paper

1. Wash your hands.

2. Explain the procedure to the client, speaking clearly, slowly, and directly. Maintain face-to-face contact whenever possible.

3. Provide privacy for the client.

4. Position the client lying straight in bed, flat on his back with arms at his sides. Be sure the bed sheet is smooth underneath the client.

5. Make a pencil mark on the sheet at the top of the head.

6. Make another mark at the client's heel (Fig. 4-84).

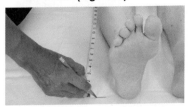

Fig. 4-84. *Make marks on the sheet at the client's head and feet.*

7. With the tape measure, measure the distance between the marks.

8. Record height.

9. Store equipment.

10. Wash your hands.

For clients who can get out of bed, you will measure height while they stand against a wall.

Equipment: tape measure, pencil, pen and paper

1. Wash your hands.

2. Explain the procedure to the client, speaking clearly, slowly, and directly. Maintain face-to-face contact whenever possible.

3. Provide privacy for the client.

4. Have the client stand with his back to the wall, with his arms at his sides and without shoes. A hard floor is better than carpet.

5. Make a pencil mark on the wall at the top of the client's head.

6. Determine the client's height. Ask client to step away. Measure the distance between the pencil mark and the floor.

7. Document the height.

8. Store equipment.

9. Wash your hands.

If it is available, you can also measure height with a standing scale for clients who can get out of bed. Help the client to step onto scale, facing away from the scale. Gently lower the measuring rod until it rests flat on the client's head. Assist the client to step off scale before recording height.

Special Procedures

Intake and Output (I&O)

The fluid a person consumes is called **intake**, or input. If a person's intake is not in a healthy range, he or she can become dehydrated. Dehydration is a serious medical condition that requires immediate attention. All fluid taken in each day cannot remain in the body. It must be eliminated as **output**. **Fluid balance** is maintaining equal input and output, or taking in and eliminating equal amounts of fluid. Most people regulate fluid balance automatically. But some clients must have their intake and output, or I&O, monitored and documented. To monitor this, you will need to measure and document all fluids the client takes by mouth, as well as all urine and vomitus the client produces.

To document intake and output, some agencies use a special form. This is called an Intake/Output (I&O) sheet. Use this form if your employer provides it. Otherwise, make your own I&O sheet on regular paper.

Conversions

A milliliter (mL or ml) is a unit of measure equal to one cubic centimeter (cc). Follow your agency's policies on whether to document using "mL" or "cc."

1 oz. = 30 mL or 30 cc

2 oz. = 60 mL

3 oz. = 90 mL

4 oz. = 120 mL

5 oz. = 150 mL

6 oz. = 180 mL

7 oz. = 210 mL

8 oz. = 240 mL

¼ cup = 2 oz. = 60 mL

½ cup = 4 oz. = 120 mL

1 cup = 8 oz. = 240 mL

Measuring and recording intake and output

Monitoring fluid balance begins with measuring intake.

Equipment: I&O sheet, graduate (measuring container, pen and paper

1. Wash your hands.

2. Explain the procedure to the client, speaking clearly, slowly, and directly. Maintain face-to-face contact whenever possible.

3. Provide privacy for the client.

4. Using the measuring container, measure the amount of fluid a client is served. Note the amount on paper, not in the visit notes.

5. When client has finished a meal or snack, measure any leftover fluids. Note this amount on paper.

6. Subtract the leftover amount from the amount served. If you have measured in ounces, convert to milliliters (mL) by multiplying by 30.

7. Document the amount of fluid consumed (in mL) in the visit notes and/or I&O record, as well as the time and what fluid was taken. Report anything unusual that was observed, such as the client refusing to drink, drinking very little, being nauseated, etc.

Measuring output is the other half of monitoring fluid balance.

Equipment: I&O sheet, graduate, gloves, pen and paper

1. Wash your hands.

2. Explain the procedure to the client, speaking clearly, slowly, and directly. Maintain face-to-face contact whenever possible.

3. Provide privacy for the client.

4. Put on gloves before handling a bedpan or urinal.

5. Pour the contents of the bedpan or urinal into the measuring container. Do not spill or splash any of the urine.

6. Measure the amount of urine at eye level on a flat surface. Note the amount on paper, converting to mL if necessary.

7. After measuring urine, empty measuring container into toilet without splashing.

8. Rinse measuring container and pour rinse water into the toilet. Clean the container and store.

9. Rinse bedpan/urinal and pour rinse water into the toilet. Clean container and store.

10. Remove and discard gloves.

11. Wash your hands before recording output.

12. Document the time and amount of urine in output column on sheet. For example: 3:45pm 200 mL urine.

Emesis, or vomiting, must be documented. It may be a sign of illness or of a reaction to medication. Some clients, such as those with cancer undergoing chemotherapy, may vomit frequently as a result of treatment. Vomiting is unpleasant. Handle it calmly. Provide comfort to the client.

To measure vomitus, pour from basin into measuring container, then discard in the toilet. If client vomits on the bed or floor, estimate the amount. Document emesis and amount in the visit notes and/or I&O sheet.

Observing, reporting and documenting emesis

Because you may not know when a client is going to vomit, you may not have time to explain what you will do and assemble supplies ahead of time. Talk to the client soothingly as you help him clean up. Tell him what you are doing to help him.

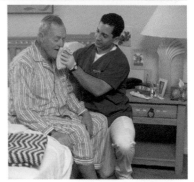

1. Put on gloves when client has vomited.

2. Provide a basin and remove it when vomiting has stopped.

3. Remove soiled linens or clothes. Set aside for launder-ing. Replace with fresh linens or clothes.

Fig. 4-85. Be calm and comforting when helping a client who has vomited.

4. If client's I&O is being moni-tored, measure and note amount of vomitus.

5. Flush vomit down the toilet. Wash and store basin.

6. Remove and discard gloves.

7. Wash your hands.

8. Put on fresh gloves.

9. Provide comfort to client: wipe face and mouth, position com-fortably, offer a sip of water or oral care (Fig. 4-85).

10. Launder soiled linens and clothes promptly in hot water.

11. Remove and discard gloves.

12. Wash your hands again.

13. Document time, amount, color, and consistency of vomitus. Look for blood in vomitus, blood-tinged vomitus, or vomi-tus that looks like wet coffee grounds.

14. Report to your supervisor immediately and get instruc-tions for diet.

Catheter Care

A **catheter** is a thin tube inserted into the body that is used to drain flu-ids or inject fluids. A urinary catheter is used to drain urine from the bladder. A straight catheter does not remain inside the body. It is removed immediately after urine is drained. An indwelling catheter remains inside the bladder for a period of time. The urine drains into a bag. An external, or condom, catheter has an attachment on the end that fits onto the penis. The external catheter is changed daily or as needed.

Guidelines: Working with Clients Who Have Catheters

G   The drainage bag must always be kept lower than the hips or bladder.

G   Keep the drainage bag off the floor.

G   Tubing should be kept as straight as possible and should not be kinked.

G   The genital area must be kept clean to prevent infection. Because the catheter goes all the way into the bladder, bacteria can enter the bladder more easily. Daily care of the genital area is especially important.

Observing and Reporting: Catheter Care

Report any of these to your supervisor:

O/R   Blood in the urine or any other unusual appearance

O/R   Catheter bag does not fill after several hours

O/R   Catheter bag fills suddenly

O/R   Catheter is not in place

O/R   Urine leaks from the catheter

O/R   Client reports pain or pressure

O/R   Odor

Many clients can clean the catheter site themselves. If you need to provide this care for a client, follow the steps below.

Providing catheter care

Equipment: bath blanket, protective pad, bath basin, bath thermometer, soap, 2-4 washcloths or wipes, 1 towel, gloves

1. Wash your hands.

2. Explain the procedure to the client, speaking clearly, slowly, and directly. Maintain face-to-face contact whenever possible.

3. Provide privacy for the client.

4. If the bed is adjustable, adjust bed to a safe working level, usually waist high. If bed is movable, lock bed wheels.

5. Lower head of bed. Position client lying flat on her back.

6. Remove or fold back top bedding, keeping client covered with bath blanket.

7. Test water temperature with thermometer or your wrist and ensure it is safe. Water temperature should be 105°F. Have client check water temperature. Adjust if necessary.

8. Put on gloves.

9. Ask the client to flex her knees and raise the buttocks off the

bed by pushing against the mattress with her feet. Place a clean protective pad under her buttocks.

10. Expose only the area necessary to clean the catheter.

11. Place towel or pad under catheter tubing before washing.

12. Apply soap to a wet washcloth. Clean area around meatus. Use a clean area of the washcloth for each stroke.

13. Hold catheter near meatus to avoid tugging the catheter.

14. Clean at least four inches of catheter nearest meatus. Move in only one direction, away from meatus. Use a clean area of the cloth for each stroke.

15. Dip a clean washcloth in the water. Rinse area around meatus, using a clean area of washcloth for each stroke.

16. Dip a clean washcloth in the water. Rinse at least four inches of catheter nearest meatus.

Move in only one direction, away from meatus (Fig. 4-86). Use a clean area of the cloth for each stroke.

17. With towel, dry at least four inches of catheter nearest meatus. Move in only one direction, away from meatus. Use a clean area of the cloth for each stroke.

18. Remove towel or pad from under the catheter tubing. Replace top covers and remove bath blanket.

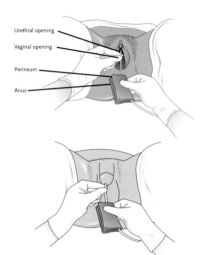

Urethral opening
Vaginal opening
Perineum
Anus

Fig. 4-86. Hold the catheter near the meatus, so that you do not tug it. Moving in only one direction, away from meatus, helps prevent infection.

19. Empty the water into the toilet. Dispose of linen in proper containers.

20. Remove and discard gloves.

21. Wash your hands.

22. Help the client dress. Arrange covers. Check that the catheter tubing is free from kinks and twists and that it is securely taped to the leg.

23. If you raised an adjustable bed, be sure to return it to its lowest position.

24. Wash your hands again.

25. Document procedure and any observations.

Emptying the catheter drainage bag

Equipment: graduate (measuring container), alcohol wipes, paper towels, gloves

1. Wash your hands.

2. Explain the procedure to the client, speaking clearly, slowly, and directly. Maintain face-to-face contact whenever possible.

3. Put on gloves.

4. Place paper towel on the floor under the drainage bag. Place measuring container on the paper towel.

5. Open the drain or spout on the bag so that urine flows out of the bag into the measuring container (Fig. 4-87). Do not let spout touch the measuring container.

6. When urine has drained, close spout. Using alcohol wipe, clean the drain spout. Replace the drain in its holder on the bag.

7. Mentally note the amount and the appearance of the urine. Empty into toilet.

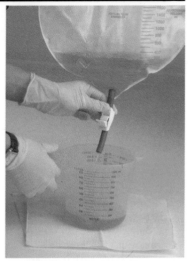

Fig. 4-87. Keep the spout from touching the graduate while draining urine.

8. Clean and store measuring container.

9. Remove and discard gloves.

10. Wash your hands.

11. Document procedure and amount of urine.

Ostomy Care

An **ostomy** is an operation to create an opening from an area inside the body to the outside. The terms "**colostomy**" and "ileostomy" refer to the surgical removal of a portion of the intestines. It may be necessary due to bowel disease, cancer, or trauma. In a client with one of these ostomies, the end of the intestine is brought out of the body through an artificial opening in the abdomen. This opening is called a **stoma**. Stool, or feces, are eliminated through the ostomy rather than through the anus.

The terms "colostomy" and "ileostomy" tell what part of the intestine was removed and the type of stool that will be eliminated. In a colostomy, stool will generally be semi-solid. With an ileostomy, stool may be liquid. It may be irritating to the skin. Clients who have had an ostomy wear a disposable bag that fits over the stoma to collect the feces. The bag is attached to the skin by adhesive. A belt may also be used to secure it.

Many people manage the ostomy appliance by themselves. If you are providing ostomy care, give careful skin care. Empty and clean or replace the ostomy bag whenever a stool is eliminated. Always wear gloves and wash hands carefully. Teach proper handwashing to clients with ostomies.

Many clients with ostomies feel they have lost control of a basic bodily function. They may be embarrassed or angry about the ostomy. Be sensitive and supportive. Always provide privacy for ostomy care.

Providing ostomy care

Equipment: disposable bed protector, bath blanket, clean ostomy bag and belt/appliance, toilet paper or gauze squares, basin of warm water, soap or cleanser, washcloth, skin cream as ordered, 2 towels, plastic disposable bag, 2 pairs of gloves

1. Wash your hands.

2. Explain the procedure to the client, speaking clearly, slowly, and directly. Maintain face-to-face contact whenever possible.

3. Provide privacy for the client.

4. If the bed is adjustable, adjust bed to a safe working level, usually waist high. If bed is movable, lock bed wheels.

5. Place bed protector under client. Cover client with a bath blanket. Pull down the top sheet and blankets. Only expose the ostomy site. Offer client a towel to keep clothing dry.

6. Put on gloves.

7. Remove ostomy bag carefully. Place it in the plastic bag. Note the color, odor, consistency, and amount of stool in the bag.

8. Wipe the area around the stoma with toilet paper or gauze squares. Discard paper/gauze in plastic bag.

9. Using a washcloth and warm soapy water, wash the area in one direction, away from the stoma (Fig. 4-88). Pat dry with another towel. Apply cream as ordered.

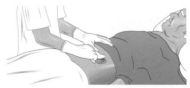

Fig. 4-88. Wash away from the stoma.

10. Place the clean ostomy appliance on client. Make sure the bottom of the bag is clamped.

11. Remove disposable bed protector and discard. Place soiled linens in proper containers.

12. Remove bag and discard in proper container.

13. Remove and discard gloves. Wash your hands.

14. Make the client comfortable. Put on fresh gloves and change linens if necessary. Cover the client and remove bath blanket and towel.

15. Return bed to lowest position if adjusted.

16. Document procedure and any observations. Note: Call your supervisor if stoma appears very red or blue, or if swelling or bleeding is present.

Collecting Specimens

Sometimes you may be asked to collect a specimen from a client. A **specimen** is a sample that is used for analysis in order to try to make a diagnosis. You may be asked to collect these different types of specimens:

- Sputum (mucus coughed up from the lungs)
- Stool (feces)
- Urine (routine, clean catch/mid-stream, or 24-hour)

Some clients will be able to collect their own specimens. Others will need your help. Be sure to explain exactly how the specimen must be collected.

Sputum specimens may help diagnose respiratory problems, illness, or evaluate the effects of medication. Early morning is the best time to collect sputum. The client should cough up the sputum and spit it directly into the specimen container.

Collecting a sputum specimen

Equipment: specimen container and lid with label (labeled with client's name, address, date and time), tissues, plastic bag, gloves, mask

1. Wash your hands.

2. Explain the procedure to the client, speaking clearly, slowly, and directly. Maintain face-to-face contact whenever possible.

3. Provide privacy for the client.

4. Put on mask and gloves. If the client has known or suspected tuberculosis or another infectious disease, you should wear a mask when collecting a sputum specimen. Coughing is one way TB bacteria can enter the air. Stand behind the client if the client can hold the specimen container by himself.

5. Ask the client to cough deeply, so that sputum comes up from the lungs. To prevent the spread of infectious material, give the client tissues to cover his mouth while coughing. Ask the client to spit the sputum into the specimen container.

6. When you have obtained a good sample (about two tablespoons of sputum), cover the container tightly. Wipe any sputum off the outside of the container with tissues. Discard the tissues. Put the specimen container in the plastic bag and seal.

7. Remove and discard gloves and mask.

8. Wash your hands.

9. Document the procedure.

Stool (feces) specimens are collected so that the stool can be tested for blood, pathogens, and other things, such as worms or amoebas. Ask the client to let you know when he or she can have a bowel movement. Be ready to collect the specimen.

Collecting a stool specimen

Equipment: specimen container and lid with label (labeled with client's name, address, date and time), 2 tongue blades, 2 pairs of gloves, bedpan (if client cannot use a portable commode or toilet), "hat" for toilet (if client can get to the bathroom), 2 plastic bags, toilet tissue, washcloth or towel, supplies for perineal care, pen

1. Wash your hands.

2. Explain the procedure to the client, speaking clearly, slowly, and directly. Maintain face-to-face contact whenever possible.

3. Provide privacy for the client.

4. Put on gloves.

5. When the client is ready to move bowels, ask him not to urinate at the same time and not to put toilet paper in with the sample. Provide a plastic bag to discard toilet paper separately.

6. Fit hat to toilet or commode, or provide client with bedpan. Leave the room and ask the client to call you when he is finished with the bowel movement.

7. Remove and discard gloves. Wash your hands. Leave the room.

8. When called, return to room. Put on clean gloves.

9. Help as necessary with perineal care. Help client wash his or her hands at the sink or using the washcloth and towel. Make the client comfortable.

10. Using the two tongue blades, take about two tablespoons of stool and put it in the container. Without touching the inside of the container, cover it tightly. Place the container in a clean plastic bag.

11. Wrap the tongue blades in toilet paper. Put them in plastic bag with used toilet paper. Discard bag in proper container. Empty the bedpan or container into the toilet. Clean and store the equipment.

12. Remove and discard gloves.

13. Wash your hands.

14. Document the procedure. Note amount and characteristics of stool.

Collecting a routine urine specimen

Equipment: urine specimen container and lid with label (labeled with client's name, address, date and time), gloves, bedpan or urinal (if client cannot use a portable commode or toilet), "hat" for toilet (if client can get to the bathroom), 2 plastic bags, washcloth, towel, paper towel, supplies for perineal care, pen

1. Wash your hands.

2. Explain the procedure to the client, speaking clearly, slowly, and directly. Maintain face-to-face contact whenever possible.

3. Provide privacy for the client.

4. Put on gloves.

5. Assist the client to the bathroom or commode, or offer the bedpan or urinal.

6. Have client void into "hat," urinal, or bedpan. Ask the client not to put toilet paper in with the sample. Provide a plastic

bag to discard toilet paper separately.

7. After urination, help as necessary with perineal care. Help client wash his hands at the sink or using the washcloth and towel. Make the client comfortable.

8. Take bedpan, urinal, or commode pail to the bathroom.

9. Pour urine into the specimen container. Specimen container should be at least half full.

10. Cover the urine container with its lid. Do not touch the inside of container. Wipe off the outside with a paper towel.

11. Place the container in a plastic bag.

12. If using a bedpan or urinal, discard extra urine. Rinse and clean equipment, and store.

13. Remove and discard gloves.

14. Wash your hands.

15. Document the procedure. Note amount and characteristics of urine.

Collecting a clean catch (mid-stream) urine specimen

Equipment: specimen kit with container, label (labeled with client's name, address, date and time), cleansing solution, gauze or towelettes, gloves, bedpan or urinal (if client cannot use the bathroom), plastic bag, washcloth, paper towel, towel, supplies for perineal care, pen

1. Wash your hands.

2. Explain the procedure to the client, speaking clearly, slowly, and directly. Maintain face-to-face contact whenever possible.

3. Provide privacy for the client.

4. Put on gloves.

5. Open the specimen kit. Do not touch the inside of the container or the inside of the lid.

6. If client cannot clean his or her perineal area, you will need to do it. See bed bath procedure earlier in this chapter for reminder on how to give perineal care.

7. Ask the client to urinate into the bedpan, urinal, or toilet, and to stop before urination is complete.

8. Place the container under the urine stream and have the client start urinating again. Fill the container at least half full. Have the client finish urinating in bedpan, urinal, or toilet.

9. Cover the urine container with its lid. Do not touch the inside of container. Wipe off the outside with a paper towel.

10. Place the container in a plastic bag.

11. After urination, help as necessary with perineal care.

12. If using a bedpan or urinal, discard extra urine. Rinse and clean equipment, and store.

13. Remove and discard gloves. Wash your hands. Help client wash his hands at the sink or using the washcloth.

14. Document the procedure. Note amount and characteristics of urine.

When collecting a 24-hour urine specimen, you will probably not be present during all 24 hours of the test. It is important to explain the collection fully to the client and family members beforehand.

Collecting a 24-hour urine specimen

Equipment: container for urine—gallon bottle or a container with lid from the lab, bedpan or urinal (for clients confined to bed), "hat" for toilet (if client can get to the bathroom), bucket of ice (if the urine must be kept cold) or a clearly-marked container can also be put in the refrigerator, funnel (if the container opening is small), gloves, washcloth or towel, supplies for perineal care, pen

1. Wash your hands.

2. Explain the procedure to the client, speaking clearly, slowly, and directly. Maintain face-to-face contact whenever possible.

3. Provide privacy for the client.

4. When beginning the collection, have the client completely empty the bladder. Discard the urine and note the exact time of this voiding. The collection will run until the same time tomorrow.

5. Label the container with client's name, address, and dates and times the collection period began and ended.

6. Put on gloves each time the client voids.

7. Pour urine from bedpan, urinal, or "hat" into the container, using the funnel as needed.

8. After each voiding, assist as necessary with perineal care. Help the client wash his hands using the washcloth and towel after each voiding.

9. Be sure the client or a family member understands that all urine is to be saved, even when you are gone. Show them how to pour the urine into the container. Remind them to store the container in the bucket of ice or in the refrigerator if ordered.

10. Clean equipment after each voiding.

11. Remove and discard gloves.

12. Wash your hands.

13. Document the time of the last void before the 24-hour collection period began, and the last void of the 24-hour collection period.

Non-Sterile Dressings

Sterile dressings are those that cover open or draining wounds. A nurse changes these dressings. Non-sterile dressings are applied to dry, closed wounds that have less chance of infection. Home health aides may assist with non-sterile dressing changes.

Changing a dry dressing using non-sterile technique

Equipment: package of square gauze dressings, adhesive tape, scissors, 2 pairs of gloves, waste bag

1. Wash your hands.

2. Explain the procedure to the client, speaking clearly, slowly, and directly. Maintain face-to-face contact whenever possible.

3. Provide privacy for the client.

4. Cut pieces of tape long enough to secure the dressing. Hang tape on the edge of a table within reach. Open the four-inch gauze square package without touching the gauze.

   Place the opened package on a flat surface.

5. Put on gloves.

6. Remove soiled dressing by gently peeling tape toward the wound. Lift dressing off the wound. Do not drag it over the wound. Observe the dressing for odor or drainage. Notice the color and size of the wound.

Dispose of used dressing in the waste bag. Remove your gloves. Place them in the waste bag.

7. Put on new gloves. Touching only outer edges of new four-inch gauze, remove it from package. Apply it to the wound. Tape gauze in place. Secure it firmly (Fig. 4-89).

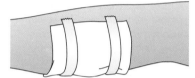

Fig. 4-89. Tape gauze in place to secure the dressing. Do not completely cover all areas of the dressing with tape.

8. Remove and discard gloves in the waste bag.

9. Wash your hands.

10. Document the procedure and your observations.

Warm and Cold Applications

Applying heat or cold to injured areas can have several good effects. Heat tends to relieve pain and muscular tension. It reduces swelling, elevates the temperature in the tissues, and increases blood flow. Increased blood flow brings more oxygen and nutrients to the tissues for healing. Cold applications can help stop bleeding. They reduce swelling and pain, and bring down high fevers.

Warm and cold applications may be dry or moist. Moisture strengthens the effect of heat and cold. This means that moist applications are more likely to cause injury. Paralysis, numbness, disorientation, confusion, dementia, and other conditions may cause a person not to be able to feel, notice, or understand damage that is occurring from a warm or cold application. Be careful when using these applications. Know how long it should be performed. Use the correct temperature as given in the care plan. Check on the application as directed.

Never perform a procedure you are not trained to do. Only perform procedures that are assigned to you.

Observing and Reporting: Warm and Cold Applications

Report the following to your supervisor:

O/R   Excessive redness

O/R   Pain

O/R   Blisters

O/R   Numbness

If you observe these signs, the application may be causing tissue damage.

Electric heating pads can also be used as heat applications. Follow the care plan. Do not use a heating pad unless it has been ordered in the care plan or by your supervisor.

Guidelines: Electric Heating Pad

G   Check the skin frequently for redness or pain. Electric heating pads do not cool down. Having it just a little too hot can be very dangerous for the client.

G   Make sure any electric heating pad you use is in good shape. Do not use it if the cord is frayed or if wires are exposed.

G   Do not use a pin to fasten the pad. The pin could contact a wire inside the pad and cause a shock.

G   Do not allow the client to lie on top of an electric heating pad.

G   Do not allow the client to use an electric heating pad near a source of water.

Applying warm compresses

Equipment: washcloth or compress, plastic wrap, towel, basin, bath thermometer

1. Wash your hands.
2. Explain the procedure to the client, speaking clearly, slowly, and directly. Maintain face-to-face contact whenever possible.
3. Provide privacy for the client.
4. Fill basin one-half to two-thirds full with hot water. Test water temperature with thermometer or your wrist and ensure it is safe. Water temperature should be no more than 105°F. Have client check water temperature. Adjust if necessary.
5. Soak the washcloth in the water and wring it out. Immediately apply it to the area needing a warm compress. Note the time. Quickly cover the washcloth with plastic wrap and the towel to keep it warm (Fig. 4-90).

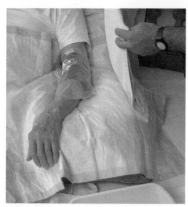

Fig. 4-90. Cover compresses to keep them warm.

6. Check the area every five minutes. Remove the compress if the area is red or numb or if the client complains of pain or discomfort. Change the compress if cooling occurs. Remove the compress after 20 minutes.

7. Commercial warm compresses are also available. If these are provided, follow the package directions and your supervisor's instructions.

8. Discard water in the toilet. Clean and store basin and other supplies. Put laundry in hamper. Discard plastic wrap.

9. Wash your hands.

10. Document the time, length, and site of procedure, and any observations.

Administering warm soaks

Equipment: basin or bathtub (depending on the area to be soaked), bath thermometer, bath blanket, towel

1. Wash your hands.

2. Explain the procedure to the client, speaking clearly, slowly, and directly. Maintain face-to-face contact whenever possible.

3. Provide privacy for the client.

4. Fill the basin or tub half full of warm water. Test water temperature with thermometer or your wrist and ensure it is safe. Water temperature should be no more than 105°F. Have client check water temperature. Adjust if necessary.

5. Immerse the body part in the basin, or help the client into the tub. Pad the edge of the basin with a towel if needed (Fig. 4-91). Use a bath blanket to cover the rest of the client if needed for extra warmth.

6. Check water temperature every five minutes. Add hot water as needed to maintain the temperature. Never add water hotter than 105°F to avoid burns. To prevent burns, tell the client not to add hot water. Observe the area for redness. Discontinue the soak if the client complains of pain or discomfort.

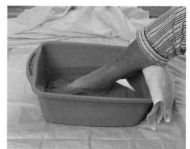

Fig. 4-91. Pad the edge of the basin to make the client more comfortable.

7. Soak for 15–20 minutes, or as ordered in the care plan.

8. Remove basin or help the client out of the tub. Use the towel to dry client.

9. Drain the tub or discard water. Clean and store basin and other supplies. Put laundry in hamper.

10. Wash your hands.

11. Document the time, length, and site of procedure. Report the client's response and any of your observations about the skin.

Another type of heat application is a sitz bath, or a warm soak of the perineal area. Sitz baths clean perineal wounds and reduce inflammation and pain. Circulation in the perineal area is increased. Voiding may be stimulated by a sitz bath. Clients with perineal swelling (such as hemorrhoids), or perineal wounds (such as those that occur during childbirth), may be ordered to take sitz baths. Because the sitz bath causes increased blood flow to the pelvic area, blood flow to other parts of the body decreases. Clients may feel weak, faint, or dizzy after a sitz bath. Always wear gloves when helping with a sitz bath.

Assisting with a sitz bath

A disposable sitz bath fits on the toilet seat and is attached to a rubber bag containing warm water (Fig. 4-92).

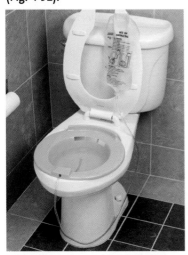

Fig. 4-92. A disposable sitz bath.
(REPRINTED WITH PERMISSION OF BRIGGS CORPORATION, 800-247-2343, WWW.BRIGGSCORP. COM)

Equipment: disposable sitz bath, bath thermometer, towels, gloves

1. Wash your hands.

2. Explain the procedure to the client, speaking clearly, slowly, and directly. Maintain face-to-face contact whenever possible.

3. Provide privacy for the client.

4. Put on gloves.

5. Fill the sitz bath two-thirds full with hot water. Place the disposable sitz bath on the toilet seat. Check the water temperature. Water temperature should be 105°F. For a sitz bath given to help relieve pain and to stimulate circulation, the water temperature may need to be higher. Follow instructions in the care plan.

6. Help the client undress and be seated on the sitz bath. A valve on the tubing connected to the bag allows the client or you to replenish the water in the sitz bath with hot water.

7. You may be required to stay with the client for safety rea-

sons. If you leave the room, check on the client every five minutes to make sure he or she is not dizzy or weak. Stay with a client who seems unsteady.

8. Assist the client out of the sitz bath in 20 minutes. Provide towels and help with dressing if needed.

9. Clean and store supplies.

10. Remove and discard gloves.

11. Wash your hands.

12. Document the procedure, including the time started and ended, the client's response, and the water temperature.

Applying ice packs

Equipment: ice pack or sealable plastic bag and crushed ice, towel to cover pack or bag

1. Wash your hands.

2. Explain the procedure to the client, speaking clearly, slowly, and directly. Maintain face-to-face contact whenever possible.

3. Provide privacy for the client.

4. Fill plastic bag or ice pack 1/2 to 2/3 full with ice. Seal bag. Remove excess air. Cover bag or ice pack with towel.

5. Apply bag to the area as ordered (Fig. 4-93). Note the time. Use another towel to cover bag if it is too cold.

6. Check the area after ten minutes for blisters, pale, white, or gray skin. Stop treatment if client complains of numbness or pain.

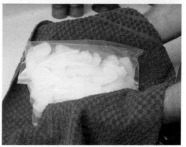

Fig. 4-93. Seal the bag filled with ice and cover it with a towel.

7. Remove ice after 20 minutes or as ordered in the care plan.

8. Return ice bag or pack to freezer.

9. Wash your hands.

10. Document the time, length, and site of procedure. Report the client's response and any of your observations about the skin.

Applying cold compresses

Equipment: basin filled with water and ice, 2 washcloths, disposable bed protector, towels

1. Wash your hands.

2. Explain the procedure to the client, speaking clearly, slowly, and directly. Maintain face-to-face contact whenever possible.

3. Provide privacy for the client.

4. Position client on plastic sheet. Rinse washcloth in basin and wring out. Cover the area to be treated with a cloth sheet or

towel. Apply cold washcloth to the area as directed (Fig. 4-94). Change washcloths often to keep area cold.

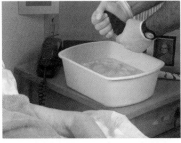

Fig. 4-94. *Wring out the washcloth before applying it to the area to be treated.*

5. Check the area after five minutes for blisters, pale, white, or gray skin. Stop treatment if client complains of numbness or pain.

6. Remove compresses after 20 minutes or as ordered in the care plan. Give client towels as needed to dry the area.

7. Clean and store basin.

8. Wash your hands.

9. Document the time, length, and site of procedure. Report the client's response and any observations about the skin.

Medications

People who need home care often need medications. HHAs do not usually handle or give medications. However, you need to understand the kinds of medicine your clients may be taking. You also need to know what to do if a client experiences side effects or refuses to take medication. If your client is taking medications that can be purchased over-the-counter (OTC) or without a physician's prescription, notify the supervisor. Sometimes OTC medications interfere with the desired effects of prescription medications.

Many states have passed different laws regarding the responsibilities and limitations for helping clients with medications. Be familiar with the regulations in your state. Provide only the assistance that is allowed.

Guidelines: Safe and Proper Use of Medications

G   Never handle or give medications unless specifically trained and assigned to do so. Do not touch the inside of a medicine bottle or the pills or other medicines themselves. Do not put any medication in a client's mouth. Handling or giving medication can have serious consequences.

G   Observe clients taking their medication. Although you cannot handle or give medications, you can remind clients to take their medications. You can also bring medication containers to clients, and provide water or food as needed to take with the medication. Always observe, report, and document as appropriate.

G   Know the difference between prescription drugs and over-the-counter drugs. Antibiotics (such as penicillin), heart drugs (such as nitroglycerin), and potent pain medication (such as codeine) are examples of prescription drugs. Aspirin or cold medications, such as decongestants, are over-the-counter drugs.

G   Be aware of all medications a client is taking, both prescription and nonprescription. There are many possible side effects and interactions among medications. Watch for symptoms such as itching, trembling or shaking, anxiety, stomach ache, diarrhea, confusion, vomiting, rash, hives, or headache. Any of these symptoms could indicate a side effect or interaction. Report any of these symptoms to your supervisor.

Knowing and remembering the five "rights" of medications will help prevent mistakes.

1. The Right Client

2. The Right Medication

3. The Right Time

4. The Right Route

5. The Right Amount

If the medication label and the care plan do not agree on any of the five "rights," call your supervisor. Also, if there is not enough information, or if you have noticed another problem with the medication (for example, the client's name is not on the container), call your supervisor.

If a client shows signs of a reaction to a medication, or complains of side effects, report these right away. Your supervisor can assess whether the symptom is caused by the medication. Your responsibility is to report your observations.

Observing and Reporting: Medications

O/R   Dizziness, fainting

O/R   Nausea, vomiting

O/R   Rash, hives, itching

O/R   Difficulty breathing, swelling of throat or eyes

O/R   Drowsiness

O/R   Headache, blurred vision

O/R   Abdominal pain

O/R   Diarrhea

°/ℝ   Any other unusual sign

In addition, report any of the following problems immediately:

°/ℝ   Client refuses to take medication as directed.

°/ℝ   Client takes the wrong dose (amount) of medication.

°/ℝ   Client takes medication at the wrong time.

°/ℝ   Client takes the wrong medication.

°/ℝ   A medication container is missing or empty.

If a client has difficulty swallowing the medication, report this to your supervisor. The doctor can then make appropriate changes. Do not crush tablets or empty capsules of medications into the client's food or drinks.

If a client has a severe allergic reaction to a medication, takes the wrong dose, or takes medications together that cause complications, emergency medical treatment is necessary. Treat an overdose, whether it was accidental or intentional, as a poisoning. Call the local Poison Control number immediately. Follow their instructions. Poison Control will send paramedics or an ambulance if needed. For severe drug reactions or interactions, call 911 for emergency help. Stay with the client. Do not give any liquids, food, or other medications unless instructed to do so by emergency personnel. Notify your supervisor as soon as possible.

You may be required to assist with the proper storage of medications. Follow these guidelines for storing medications:

Guidelines: Proper Storage of Medications

G   Keep the client's medications in one place, separate from medicine used by other members of the household.

G   If there are young children or a disoriented elderly person in the home, recommend to the family that medications be locked away.

G   All medications should be kept in child-proof containers if children are in the home. To avoid an accidental overdose, keep medications out of reach of children.

G   If medicine requires refrigeration, make sure the bottle is on an upper shelf in the back, out of a child's reach.

G   All medications should be stored away from heat and light, as appropriate.

G   The client or family member should discard medications that have expired, are not labeled, or are discolored. Make sure these medications are not discarded in the trash. Children or animals may have access to them. Ask your supervisor for specific disposal instructions if the client or family will not dispose of expired medications. Do not dispose of them yourself.

Drug misuse and abuse may be accidental or deliberate. It includes the following:

- Refusing to take medications
- Taking the wrong dose or taking it at the wrong time
- Mixing medication with alcohol
- Taking drugs that have not been prescribed
- Taking illegal drugs

Misuse and abuse of drugs is extremely dangerous. It can even be fatal. Be alert to the signs of misuse or abuse and report them to your supervisor immediately.

Observing and Reporting: Drug Misuse and Abuse

O/R Depression

O/R Anorexia

O/R Change in sleep patterns

O/R Withdrawn behavior or moodiness

O/R Secrecy

O/R Verbal abusiveness

O/R Poor relationships with family members

The drugs that pose the highest risk for causing drug dependency are pain medications, tranquilizers, muscle relaxers, and sleeping pills. Substance abuse is the repeated use of legal or illegal drugs, cigarettes, or alcohol in a way that is harmful to oneself or others. A substance need not be illegal for it to be abused. Alcohol and cigarettes are legal for adults, but are often abused. Over-the-counter medications, including diet aids and decongestants, can be addictive and harmful. Even household substances such as paint or glue are sometimes abused, causing injury and death.

Report these signs to your supervisor. You can report your observations without accusing anyone of abuse. Simply report what you see, not what you think the cause may be.

Observing and Reporting: Substance Abuse

- O/R Changes in personality, moodiness, strange behavior, disruption of routines
- O/R Irritability
- O/R Changes in appearance (red eyes, dilated pupils, weight loss)
- O/R Odor of cigarettes, liquor, or other substances on breath or clothes
- O/R Diminished sense of smell
- O/R Loss of appetite
- O/R Inability to function normally
- O/R Confusion/forgetfulness
- O/R Blackouts or memory loss
- O/R Frequent accidents
- O/R Need for money, or money missing from the home
- O/R Alcohol or cigarettes missing from the home
- O/R Problems with family/friends

Oxygen

Clients may receive oxygen therapy. **Oxygen therapy** is the administration of oxygen to increase the supply of oxygen to the lungs. This increases the availability of oxygen to the body tissues. Oxygen therapy is often used to treat breathing difficulties and is prescribed by a doctor. Home health aides never stop, adjust, or administer oxygen. The agency that supplies the oxygen will service the equipment and will provide training in its use.

Oxygen will be delivered to the home in tanks or produced by an oxygen concentrator. An oxygen concentrator is a box-like device that changes air in the room into air with more oxygen. Oxygen concentrators are quiet machines. They can be larger units or portable ones that can move or travel with the client. Oxygen concentrators typically plug into wall outlets and are turned on and off by a switch. It may take a while for the oxygen concentrator to reach full power after it is turned on.

Some clients receive oxygen through a nasal cannula. A nasal cannula is a piece of plastic tubing that fits around the face and is secured by a strap that goes over the ears and around the back of the head. The face piece has two short prongs made of tubing. These prongs fit inside the nose, and oxygen is delivered through them. A respiratory therapist fits the cannula. The length of the prongs (usually no more than half an inch) is adjusted for the client's comfort. The client can talk and eat while wearing the cannula.

Clients who do not need concentrated oxygen all the time may use a face mask when they need oxygen. The face mask fits over the nose and mouth. It is secured by a strap that goes over the ears and around the back of the head. The mask should be checked to see that it fits snugly on the client's face, but it should not pinch the face. It is difficult for a client to talk when wearing an oxygen face mask. The mask must be removed for the client to eat or drink anything.

Oxygen can be irritating to the nose and mouth. The strap of a nasal cannula or face mask can also cause irritation around the ears. Wash and dry skin carefully, and provide frequent mouth care. Offer the client plenty of fluids. Report and document any irritation you observe.

Oxygen is a very dangerous fire hazard because it makes other things burn. Oxygen itself does not burn; it merely supports combustion. **Combustion** means the process of burning. Working around oxygen requires special safety precautions.

Guidelines: Working Safely Around Oxygen

G Remove all fire hazards from the area. Fire hazards include electrical shavers, hair dryers, other electrical appliances, cigarettes, matches, and flammable fluids. **Flammable** means easily ignited and capable of burning quickly. Examples of flammable liquids are alcohol and nail polish remover. Notify your supervisor if a fire hazard is present and the client does not want it removed.

G Post "No Smoking" and "Oxygen in Use" signs. Never allow smoking in the room or area where oxygen is used or stored.

G Never allow candles or other open flames around oxygen.

G Learn how to turn oxygen off in case of fire. Never adjust oxygen level.

G Report if the nasal cannula or face mask is causing skin irritation. Check behind the ears for irritation from the nasal cannula.

IVs

IV stands for **intravenous**, or into a vein. A client with an IV is receiving medication, nutrition, or fluids through a vein. When a physician prescribes an IV, a nurse inserts a needle into a vein. This allows direct access to the bloodstream. Medication, nutrition, or fluids either drip from a bag suspended on a pole or are pumped by a portable pump through a tube and into the vein. Some clients with chronic conditions may have a permanent opening for IVs. This opening has been surgically created to allow easy access for IV fluids.

HHAs never insert or remove IV lines. You will not be responsible for care of the IV site. Your only responsibility for IV care is to report and document any observations of changes or problems with the IV.

Observing and Reporting: IVs

Report any of the following to your supervisor:

- O/R The tube/needle falls out or is removed.
- O/R The tubing disconnects.
- O/R The dressing around the IV site is loose or not intact.
- O/R Blood is visible in the tubing or around the site of the IV.
- O/R The site is swollen or discolored.
- O/R The client complains of pain.
- O/R The bag is broken, or the level of fluid does not seem to decrease.
- O/R The IV fluid is not dripping.
- O/R The IV fluid is nearly gone.
- O/R The pump beeps, indicating a problem.
- O/R The pump is dropped.

Do not do any of the following when caring for a client who has an IV:

- Take a blood pressure reading on an arm with an IV
- Get the IV site wet
- Pull or catch the tubing in anything, such as clothing
- Leave the tubing kinked
- Lower the IV bag below the IV site
- Touch the clamp
- Disconnect the IV from the pump

V.
Special Clients, Special Needs

Disabilities and Mental Illnesses

Disabilities

A disability is the impairment of a physical or mental function. Disability may result from a disease, a complication of pregnancy, or an injury. Depending on the disability, a person may not be able to perform activities of daily living (ADLs). Work and social activities may be limited. People with disabilities may be more susceptible to illness. By strictly following the client care plan and carefully observing and reporting, you can help your clients with disabilities avoid illness. Your efforts may also help clients lead more independent lives.

Families of people with disabilities may find it difficult to cope with the stress a disability can cause. They may feel resentment, disappointment, guilt or shame, and anger or frustration. Caring for someone with a disability can be a big responsibility. It affects a family's time, energy, patience, and financial resources. Home health aides can give family members a much-needed break. Clients and their families may need additional support, including counseling, to help deal with the disability. Tell your supervisor if you think a client or family member needs additional support.

Illness or disability requires clients and families to make adjustments. Making these adjustments may be difficult, depending on the family's emotional, spiritual, and financial resources. Some of the personal adjustments include the following:

- Accepting the illness or disability and its long-term consequences
- Finding money to pay expenses of hospitalization or home care
- Dealing with paperwork required for insurance, Medicaid, or Medicare
- Taking care of tasks the client can no longer handle
- Understanding medical information and making difficult care decisions
- Providing daily care when the aide cannot be there

- Caring for children while caring for an elderly loved one (called the "sandwich generation"—being "sandwiched" between two generations)

Guidelines: Working with Disabilities

G Promote self-care and independence. Help your clients with disabilities do all they can for themselves. Give them opportunities to show what they can do. Do not take over a task just because you can do it faster or better. The sense of independence, dignity, acceptance, social interaction, and self-worth are all boosted when the client is able to perform a task for himself. However, do not push a client beyond his or her abilities.

G Assure the client's safety. Be aware of accidents that commonly occur in the home. Most can be avoided if you think ahead. Think critically about each client's abilities and disabilities. Safety concerns vary depending on the disability.

G Promote the client's health and comfort. Help your clients by maintaining nutrition and hydration and by assisting with personal care. The care plan and your assignment sheet will include instructions for this type of care. To provide further comfort, watch and listen to the client.

G Maintain the client's dignity and self-worth. Treat a client who is disabled with the same respect you would give any client. Be sensitive to the client's feelings. Find ways to make your clients feel good about themselves. Allow and encourage the client to direct how and when care is provided.

G Maintain the stability of the client's household. Help maintain the stability of the household by being punctual and dependable. Respect the schedules of the family. Work cheerfully, calmly, and efficiently.

G Observe, report, and document carefully. For clients with disabilities that affect mobility, be very careful to observe and report changes in the skin. Pressure sore prevention is an important role of the home health aide. Emotional changes should also be observed and reported. Clients may be at risk for depression. Report any signs of depression, including moodiness, weight loss or gain, fatigue, or withdrawal.

Mental Illnesses

Mental health is the normal functioning of emotional and intellectual abilities. Traits of a person who is mentally healthy include the abilities to:

- Get along with others
- Adapt to change

- Care for self and others
- Give and accept love
- Deal with situations that cause anxiety, disappointment, and frustration
- Take responsibility for decisions, feelings, and actions
- Control and fulfill desires and impulses appropriately

While it involves emotional and mental functioning, mental illness is a disease. It is like any physical disease. It produces signs and symptoms and affects the body's ability to function. It responds to proper treatment and care. Mental illness disrupts a person's ability to function at a normal level in the family, home, or community. It often causes inappropriate behavior. Some signs and symptoms of mental illness include confusion, disorientation, **agitation**, and anxiety. Mental illness can be caused or made worse by chronic stress from any of these conditions:

- Physical factors, such as illness, disability, aging, substance abuse, or chemical imbalance
- Environmental factors, such as weak interpersonal or family relationships or traumatic early life experiences
- Heredity
- Stress

A fallacy is a false belief. The greatest fallacy about mental illness is that people who are mentally ill can control it. Mentally ill people cannot simply choose to be well. Mental illness is a disease like any other physical illness. Mentally healthy people are able to control their emotions and responses. Mentally ill people may not have this control. Knowing that mental illness is a disease helps you work with mentally ill clients.

Mental health is important to physical health. The ability of mentally healthy people to reduce stress can help prevent some physical illnesses. It can help them cope if illness or disability occur. Mental health can help protect and improve physical health. The reverse is also true. Physical illness or disability can cause or worsen mental illness. The stress these conditions create takes a toll on mental health.

Different types of mental illness will determine how well clients are able to communicate. Treat each client as an individual.

Guidelines: Communicating with Mentally Ill Clients

G   Do not talk to adults as if they were children.

G   Use simple, clear statements and a normal tone of voice.

G Be sure that what you say and how you say it show respect and concern.

G Sit or stand at a normal distance from the client. Be aware of your body language.

G Be honest and direct, as you would with any client.

G Avoid arguments.

G Maintain eye contact.

G Listen carefully.

There are many degrees of mental illness, from mild to severe. Being able to recognize some behaviors may make it easier to understand clients who are mentally ill.

Anxiety-Related Disorders: Anxiety is uneasiness or fear, often about a situation or condition. Physical symptoms of anxiety-related disorders include shakiness, muscle aches, sweating, cold and clammy hands, dizziness, fatigue, racing heart, cold or hot flashes, a choking or smothering sensation, and a dry mouth.

Phobias are an intense form of anxiety. Many people are very afraid of certain things (for example, dogs or snakes) or situations (like being in a confined space, or flying). For a mentally ill person, a phobia is a disabling terror. It prevents the person from participating in normal activities. Other anxiety-related disorders include panic disorder, in which a person is terrified for no known reason. Obsessive compulsive disorder is obsessive behavior a person uses to cope with anxiety. For example, a person may wash his hands over and over as a way of dealing with anxiety. Anxiety-related disorders may also be caused by a traumatic experience. This is known as post-traumatic stress disorder.

Depression: Clinical **depression** is a serious mental illness that may cause intense mental, emotional, and physical pain and disability. It also makes other illnesses worse. If untreated, it may result in suicide. Clinical depression is not a normal reaction to stress. Sadness is only one symptom of this illness. Not all people who have depression complain of sadness or appear sad. Other common symptoms of clinical depression include:

• Pain, including headaches, abdominal pain, and other body aches

• Low energy or fatigue

• Apathy, or lack of interest in activities

• Irritability

• Anxiety

- Loss of appetite or overeating
- Problems with sexual functioning and desire
- Sleeplessness, difficulty sleeping, or excessive sleeping
- Lack of attention to basic personal care tasks (e.g. bathing, combing hair, changing clothes)
- Intense feelings of despair
- Guilt
- Trouble concentrating
- Withdrawal and isolation
- Repeated thoughts of suicide and death

Schizophrenia: Contrary to popular belief, schizophrenia does not mean "split personality." **Schizophrenia** is a brain disorder that affects a person's ability to think and communicate clearly. It also affects the ability to manage emotions, make decisions, and understand reality. It affects a person's ability to interact with other people. Some of the symptoms of schizophrenia are:

- Hallucinations
- Delusions
- Disorganized thinking and speech
- Moving slowly, repeating rhythmic gestures or movements
- Showing less emotion, less interest
- Lack of energy

Guidelines: Caring for Mentally Ill Clients

G Observe clients carefully for changes in condition or abilities. Document and report your observations.

G Support the client and his family and friends. Your positive, professional attitude encourages them.

G Encourage clients to do as much for themselves as possible. Progress may be very slow. Be patient, supportive, and positive.

G Mental illness can be treated. Medication and psychotherapy are common methods. Medication must be taken properly to promote benefits and reduce side effects. Home health aides may be assigned to observe clients taking their medications. Psychotherapy is a method of treating mental illness that involves talking about one's problems with mental health professionals.

Observing and Reporting: Mentally Ill Clients

O/R   Changes in ability

O/R   Positive or negative mood changes, especially withdrawal

O/R   Behavior changes, including changes in personality, extreme behavior, and behavior that does not seem to fit the situation

O/R   Comments, even jokes, about hurting self or others

O/R   Failure to take medicine or improper use of medicine

O/R   Real or imagined physical symptoms

O/R   Events, situations, or people that seem to upset or excite clients

Special Conditions

There are certain special conditions or diseases you will see in the home that require specific types of care. Below is a quick overview of these conditions for you to use as a reference when you care for clients who have them:

- Arthritis
- Cancer
- Diabetes
- Cerebral Vascular Accident (CVA) or Stroke
- Multiple Sclerosis (MS)
- Circulatory Disorders
- HIV and AIDS
- Dementia
- Alzheimer's Disease (AD)
- Chronic Obstructive Pulmonary Disease (COPD)
- Tuberculosis (TB)
- Hip or Knee Replacement

Arthritis

Arthritis is a general term that refers to inflammation, or swelling, of the joints. It causes stiffness, pain, and decreased mobility. Arthritis may be the result of aging, injury, or an autoimmune illness. Autoimmune illnesses cause the body's immune system to attack normal tissue in the body. There are several types of arthritis.

Osteoarthritis is a common type of arthritis that affects the elderly. It may occur with aging or as the result of joint injury. Hips and knees, which are weight-bearing joints, are usually affected. Joints of the fingers, thumbs, and spine can also be affected. Pain and stiffness seem to increase in cold or damp weather.

Rheumatoid arthritis can affect people of all ages. Joints become red, swollen, and very painful. Movement is restricted. Fever, fatigue, and weight loss are also symptoms.

Arthritis is generally treated with some or all of the following:

- Anti-inflammatory medications such as aspirin or ibuprofen
- Local applications of heat to reduce swelling and pain
- Range of motion exercises
- Regular exercise and/or activity routines
- Diet to reduce weight or maintain strength

Guidelines: Caring for Clients with Arthritis

G Watch for stomach irritation or heartburn caused by aspirin or ibuprofen. Some clients cannot take these medications. Report signs of stomach irritation or heartburn immediately.

G Encourage activity. Gentle activity can help reduce the effects of arthritis. Follow the care plan instructions carefully. Use canes or other walking aids as needed.

G Adapt activities of daily living (ADLs) to allow independence. Many devices are available to help clients to bathe, dress, and feed themselves even when they have arthritis.

G Choose clothing that is easy to put on and fasten. Suggest handrails and safety bars for the bathroom. Special utensils are available to make it easier for clients to feed themselves.

G Treat each client as an individual. Arthritis is very common among elderly clients. Do not assume that all clients have the same symptoms and need the same care.

G Help maintain client's self-esteem by encouraging self-care. Have a positive attitude. Listen to the client's feelings. You can help him to be independent as long as possible.

Cancer

Cancer is a general term used to describe many types of malignant tumors. A **tumor** is a group of abnormally growing cells. Benign tumors are considered non-cancerous. They usually grow slowly in local areas. Malignant tumors are cancerous. They grow rapidly and invade surrounding tissues.

Cancer invades local tissue, and it can spread to other parts of the body. When cancer spreads from the site where it first appears, it can affect other body systems. In general, treatment is more difficult and cancer is more deadly after this has occurred. Cancer often appears first in the breast, colon, rectum, uterus, prostate, lungs, or skin. There is no known cure for cancer, but some treatments are effective.

Risk factors for cancer include the following:

- Tobacco use
- Exposure to sunlight
- Excessive alcohol use
- Exposure to some chemicals and industrial agents
- Radiation
- Poor nutrition
- Lack of physical activity

When diagnosed early, cancer can often be treated and controlled. The American Cancer Society has identified some warning signs of cancer:

- Unexplained weight loss
- Fever
- Fatigue
- Pain
- Skin changes
- Change in bowel or bladder habits
- Sores that do not heal
- Unusual bleeding or discharge
- Thickening or lump in the breast or other part of the body
- Indigestion or difficulty swallowing
- Recent change in a wart or mole
- Nagging cough or hoarseness

People with cancer can often live longer and sometimes recover if they are treated early. Often these treatments are combined:

- Surgery
- Chemotherapy
- Radiation

Guidelines: Caring for Clients with Cancer

G   Each case is different. Cancer is a general term and refers to many separate situations. Clients may live many years or only several months. Treatment affects each person differently. Do not make assumptions about a client's condition.

G   Clients may want to talk or may avoid talking. Respect each client's needs. Be honest. Never tell a client, "Everything will be okay." Be sensitive. Remember that cancer is a disease, and its cause is unknown.

G   Good nutrition is very important for clients with cancer. Follow the care plan carefully. Clients frequently have poor appetites. Encourage a variety of food and small portions. Liquid nutrition supplements may be used in addition to, not in place of, meals. If nausea or swallowing is a problem, foods such as soups, gelatin, or starches may appeal to the client. Use plastic utensils for a client receiving chemotherapy. It makes food taste better. Metal utensils cause a bitter taste.

G   Cancer can cause great pain, especially in the late stages. Watch for signs of pain. Assist with comfort measures, including back rubs, repositioning and providing conversation, music, or reading materials. Report if pain seems to be uncontrolled.

G   Use lotion regularly on dry or delicate skin. Do not apply lotion to areas receiving radiation therapy.

G   Help clients brush and floss teeth regularly. Medications, nausea, vomiting, or mouth infections may cause a bad taste in the mouth. Use a soft-bristled toothbrush and rinse with baking soda and water or a prescribed rinse. Use oral swabs, rather than toothbrushes, for clients with mouth sores. Be very gentle when giving oral care.

G   People with cancer may have a low self-image because they are weak and their appearance has changed. For example, hair loss is a common side effect of chemotherapy. Assist with grooming if desired.

G   If visitors help cheer your client, encourage visits and do not intrude. If some times of day are better than others, suggest this to the client's friends and family.

G   Caring for a person with cancer at home can be very difficult for family members. Be alert to needs that are not being met or stresses created by the illness. Report your observations.

G   Report any of the following to your supervisor:

   •   Increased weakness or fatigue

- Weight loss

- Nausea, vomiting, or diarrhea

- Changes in appetite

- Fainting

- Signs of depression

- Confusion

- Blood in stool or urine

- Change in mental status

- Changes in skin

- New lumps, sores, or rashes

- Increase in pain, or unrelieved pain

Numerous services and support groups are available for people with cancer and their families or caregivers. Hospitals, hospice programs, and religious organizations offer many resources. These include meal services, transportation to doctors' offices or hospitals, counseling, and support groups. Visit the American Cancer Society online at cancer.org, or call the local or state chapter. The National Association of Area Agencies on Aging, n4a.org, operates the Eldercare Locator, which is a free national service that links older adults and caregivers to aging information and resources in their own communities.

Diabetes

In diabetes mellitus, commonly called **diabetes**, the pancreas does not produce enough insulin or properly use insulin. Insulin is a hormone that converts glucose, or natural sugar, into energy for the body. Without insulin to process the glucose, these sugars collect in the blood. This causes problems with circulation and can damage vital organs. Diabetes commonly occurs in people with a family history of the illness, in the elderly, and in people who are obese. There are two major types of diabetes:

Type 1 diabetes is usually diagnosed in children and young adults. It was formerly known as juvenile diabetes. It most often appears before age 20. In type 1 diabetes, the body does not produce insulin. This condition will continue throughout a person's life. A person can develop type 1 diabetes up to age 40. Type 1 diabetes is treated with insulin and a special diet.

Type 2 diabetes, also called adult-onset diabetes, is the most common form of diabetes. In type 2 diabetes, either the body does not produce enough insulin or the body fails to properly use insulin. This is known as "insulin resistance." Type 2 diabetes usually develops slowly. It is the milder form of diabetes. It typically develops around age 35. Type 2 diabetes often occurs in obese people or those with a family history of the disease. It can usually be controlled with diet and/or oral medications.

People with diabetes may have these signs and symptoms:

- Excessive thirst
- Extreme hunger
- Frequent urination
- Weight loss
- High levels of blood sugar
- Sugar in the urine
- Sudden vision changes
- Tingling or numbness in hands or feet
- Feeling very tired much of the time
- Very dry skin
- Sores that are slow to heal
- More infections than usual

Diabetes can lead to further complications:

- Changes in the circulatory system can cause heart attack and stroke, reduced circulation, poor wound healing, and kidney and nerve damage.
- Damage to the eyes can cause vision loss and blindness.
- Poor circulation and impaired wound healing may cause leg and foot ulcers, infected wounds, and gangrene. Gangrene can lead to amputation.
- Insulin reaction and diabetic ketoacidosis can be serious complications of diabetes. Refer to the Medical Emergencies section for more information. Discuss each individual client's status with your supervisor.

Diabetes must be carefully controlled to prevent complications and severe illness. When working with clients with diabetes, follow care plan instructions carefully.

Guidelines: Caring for Clients with Diabetes

G   Follow diet instructions exactly. The intake of carbohydrates, including breads, potatoes, grains, pasta, and sugars, must be regulated.
Meals must be eaten at the same time each day. The client must eat
everything that is served. If a client refuses to eat what is served, or
if you suspect that he or she is not following the diet when you leave,
report this to your supervisor.

G   Encourage your client to follow his exercise program. A regular exercise program is important. Exercise affects how quickly the human
body uses food. Exercise also improves circulation. Exercises may
include walking or other active exercise. They may also include passive range of motion exercises. Assist with exercises as necessary. Be
positive. Try to make them fun.

G   Observe the client's management of insulin doses. Doses are cal-
culated exactly. They should be administered at the same time each
day. Home health aides are not permitted to inject insulin.

G   Perform urine and blood tests as directed. Sometimes the care plan
will specify a daily blood or urine test to determine sugar or insulin
levels. Not all states allow home health aides to do this. Know your
state's rules. Your agency will train you.

G   Perform foot care as directed. People with diabetes have poor circulation. Even a small sore on the leg or foot can grow into a large
wound. It can require amputation. Careful foot care, including regular inspection, is vital. The goals of diabetic foot care are to check
for signs of irritation or sores, to promote blood circulation, and to
prevent infection.

G   Encourage diabetic clients to wear comfortable, well-fitting leather
shoes that do not hurt their feet. Leather shoes breathe and help
prevent buildup of moisture. To avoid injuries to the feet, diabetics
should never go barefoot. Cotton socks are best because they absorb
sweat. Home health aides should never trim or clip any client's toenails, but especially not a diabetic client's toenails. Only a nurse or
doctor should do this.

Providing foot care for the diabetic client

*Equipment: basin of warm water,
mild soap, washcloth, soft towel,
lotion, cotton balls, cotton socks,
shoes or slippers, gloves*

1. **Wash your hands.**

2. **Explain the procedure to the
client, speaking clearly, slowly,
and directly. Maintain face-to-
face contact whenever possible.**

3. **Provide privacy for the client.**

4. Put on gloves.

5. Using the washcloth and soap, wash the feet gently. Rinse with the warm water.

6. Gently pat the feet dry, wiping between the toes.

7. Starting at the toes and working up to the ankles, gently rub lotion into the feet with circular strokes. Your goal is to increase circulation, so take several minutes on each foot. Do not put lotion between the toes.

8. Observe the feet, ankles, and legs for dry skin, irritation, blisters, redness, sores, corns, discoloration, or swelling.

9. Help client put on socks and shoes or slippers.

10. Put used linens in the laundry. Pour water into the toilet. Clean and store basin and supplies.

11. Remove and discard gloves.

12. Wash your hands.

13. Document the procedure, including any abnormalities you observed on the feet or legs.

People with diabetes must be very careful about what they eat. To keep their blood glucose levels near normal, they must eat the right amount of the right type of food at the right time. To make it easier to keep track of what they should eat, diabetics often follow meal plans and use exchange lists.

A dietitian, working with the client, creates a meal plan that includes all the right types and amounts of food for each day. Then the client uses exchange lists, or lists of similar foods that can be substituted for one another, to make up a menu. For example, the meal plan might call for one starch and one fruit to be eaten as a snack. Looking at the exchange list, the client may choose which starch and fruit he wants to eat. The equivalent serving size for each food is also given, so the person will get the right amount of carbohydrates, protein, and fat to meet his or her requirements. Using meal plans and exchange lists, a person with diabetes can control his diet while still making his own food choices. You will not be responsible for making up meal plans. A dietitian will create meal plans, provide exchange lists, and train the client to use them. If you are assigned to prepare food for the client, however, you should follow the diet exactly. Refer to the "Special Diets" section in Section VI for more information.

CVA or Stroke

The medical term for a stroke is a cerebrovascular accident (CVA). CVA, or stroke, is caused when blood supply to the brain is cut off suddenly by a clot or a ruptured blood vessel. Without blood, part of the brain gets no oxygen. This causes brain cells to die. Refer to the Medical Emergencies section for more information on the warning signs of a stroke.

Strokes can be mild or severe. After a stroke, a person may experience any of these problems:

- Paralysis on one side of the body, called **hemiplegia**
- Weakness on one side of the body, called **hemiparesis**
- Inability to speak or speak clearly, called **expressive aphasia**
- Inability to understand spoken or written words, called **receptive aphasia**
- Loss of sensations such as temperature or touch
- Loss of bowel or bladder control
- Confusion
- Poor judgment
- Memory loss
- Loss of cognitive abilities
- Tendency to ignore one side of the body, called one-sided neglect
- Laughing or crying without any reason, or when it is inappropriate, called **emotional lability**
- Difficulty swallowing, called **dysphagia**

The two sides of the brain control different functions. Symptoms depend on which side of the brain the stroke affected. Weaknesses on the right side of the body indicate that the left side of the brain was affected. Weaknesses on the left side of the body indicate that the right side of the brain was affected.

If the stroke was mild, the client may experience few, if any, of these effects. Physical therapy may help restore physical abilities. Speech and occupational therapy can also help with communication and performing ADLs.

Guidelines: Caring for Clients Recovering from Stroke

G   Clients with paralysis, weakness, or loss of movement will usually receive physical or occupational therapy. Clients may also need to perform leg exercises to improve circulation. Safety is important when post-CVA clients are exercising. Assist carefully with exercises as ordered.

G   Never refer to the weaker side as the "bad side," or talk about the "bad" leg or arm. Use the terms "weaker," "affected," or "involved" to refer to the side with paralysis

G   Clients with speech loss or communication problems may receive speech therapy. You may be asked to help. This includes helping clients to recognize written words or spoken words. Speech therapists will also evaluate a client's swallowing ability. They will decide if swallowing therapy or thickened liquids are needed.

G   Experiencing confusion or memory loss is upsetting. People often cry for no apparent reason after suffering a stroke. Be patient and understanding. Keeping a routine may help clients feel more secure.

G   Encourage independence and self-esteem. Let the client do things for him- or herself whenever possible, even if you could do a better or faster job. Make tasks less difficult for clients. Appreciate and acknowledge clients' efforts to do things for themselves even when they are unsuccessful. Praise even the smallest successes to build confidence.

G   Always check on the client's body alignment. Sometimes an arm or leg can be caught and the client is unaware.

G   Pay special attention to skin care and observe for changes in the skin if a client is unable to move.

G   If clients have a loss of touch or sensation, check for potentially harmful situations (for example, heat and sharp objects). If clients are unable to sense or move part of the body, check and change positioning to prevent pressure sores.

G   Adapt procedures when providing personal care for clients with one-sided paralysis or weakness.

G   When helping with transfers or walking, stand on the weaker side. Always use a gait belt for safety. Support the weaker side and lead with the stronger side.

When assisting with dressing, remember to:

G   Dress the weaker side first. Place the weaker arm or leg into the clothing. This prevents unnecessary bending and stretching of the limb. Undress the stronger side first. Then remove the weaker arm or leg from clothing to prevent the limb from being stretched and twisted.

G   Use assistive equipment to help the client dress himself. Encourage self-care.

When assisting with communication, remember to:

G   Keep your questions and directions simple.

G   Phrase questions so they can be answered with a "yes" or "no."

G   Agree on signals, such as shaking or nodding the head, or raising a hand or finger to indicate "yes" or "no."

G   Give clients time to respond. Listen attentively.

G   Use a pencil and paper if a client is able to write. A thick handle or tape wrapped around the pen may help the client hold it more easily.

G   Use verbal and nonverbal communication to express your positive attitude. Let the client know you have confidence in his or her abilities through smiles, touches, and gestures.

G   Use pictures, gestures, or pointing. Use communication boards or special cards to make communication easier.

G   Keep a bell or other call signal within reach of clients. They can let you know when you are needed.

G   Never talk about a client as if he or she were not there. Speak to all clients with respect.

When assisting with eating, remember to:

G   Be sure to place food in the client's field of vision.

G   Use assistive devices such as silverware with built-up handle grips, plate guards, and drinking cups.

G   Watch for signs of choking.

G   Serve soft foods if swallowing is difficult.

G   Always place food in the unaffected, or non-paralyzed, side of the mouth.

G   Make sure food is swallowed before offering more bites.

Monitoring the home safety of clients who have had a stroke is essential. Clients who are unsteady, weak, or confused are at risk of falling. Clients with loss of sensation are at risk of burning themselves in the bathroom or at the stove. Some safety tips include:

• Remove any hazards from the home, including unnecessary clutter or throw rugs.

• Unplug appliances like toasters and coffee makers when not in use.

• Check the refrigerator and cabinets for spoiled food. A stroke may impair the senses of smell and taste.

• Report any suspected safety hazards to your supervisor.

Multiple Sclerosis (MS)

Multiple sclerosis (MS) is a progressive disease that affects the central nervous system. When a person has MS, the protective covering for the nerves, spinal cord, and white matter of the brain breaks down over time.

Without this covering, or sheath, nerves cannot send messages to and from the brain in a normal way. People with MS have varying abilities. Multiple sclerosis is usually diagnosed when a person is in his or her early twenties to thirties. It progresses slowly and unpredictably. Symptoms include blurred vision, fatigue, tremors, poor balance, and trouble walking. Weakness, numbness, tingling, incontinence, and behavior changes are also symptoms. MS can cause blindness, contractures, and loss of function in the arms and legs.

Guidelines: Caring for Clients with Multiple Sclerosis

G   Assist with ADLs as needed. Be patient with self-care and movement. Allow enough time for tasks. Offer rest periods as necessary.

G   Give client plenty of time to communicate. People with MS may have trouble forming their thoughts. Be patient and do not rush them.

G   Prevent falls, which may be due to a lack of coordination, fatigue, or vision problems.

G   Stress can worsen the effects of MS. Be calm. Listen to clients when they want to talk.

G   Encourage a healthy diet with plenty of fluids.

G   Give regular skin care to prevent pressure sores.

G   Assist with range of motion exercises to prevent contractures and to strengthen muscles.

Circulatory Disorders

Hypertension or High Blood Pressure

When blood pressure is consistently 140/90 or higher, a person is diagnosed as having **hypertension**, or high blood pressure. If blood pressure is between 120/80 and 139/89 mmHg, it is called prehypertension. This means that the person does not have high blood pressure now but is likely to develop it in the future. Hypertension is caused by atherosclerosis, or a hardening and narrowing of the blood vessels. It can also result from kidney disease, tumors of the adrenal gland, and pregnancy. Hypertension can develop in persons of any age.

Signs and symptoms of hypertension are not always obvious, especially in the early stages. Often it is only discovered when a blood pressure measurement is taken. Persons with the disease may complain of headache, blurred vision, and dizziness.

Guidelines: Caring for Clients with Hypertension

G   Hypertension can lead to serious problems such as CVA, heart attack, kidney disease, or blindness. Treatment to control it is vital. Clients may take medication that lowers cholesterol or diuretics. Diuretics are drugs that reduce fluid in the body.

G   Clients may also have a prescribed exercise program or be on a special low-fat, low-sodium diet. Encourage clients to follow their diet and exercise programs.

Coronary Artery Disease (CAD)

Coronary artery disease occurs when the blood vessels in the coronary arteries narrow. This reduces the supply of blood to the heart muscle and deprives it of oxygen and nutrients. Over time, as fatty deposits block the artery, the muscle that was supplied by the blood vessel dies. CAD can lead to heart attack or stroke.

The heart muscle that is not getting enough oxygen causes chest pain, pressure, or discomfort, called **angina pectoris**. The heart needs more oxygen during exercise, stress, excitement, or a heavy meal. In CAD, narrowed blood vessels prevent the extra blood with oxygen from getting to the heart.

The pain of angina pectoris is usually described as pressure or tightness in the left side of the chest or in the center of the chest behind the sternum or breastbone. Some people complain of the pain radiating or extending down the inside of the left arm or to the neck and left side of the jaw. A person suffering from angina pectoris may perspire or appear pale. The person may feel dizzy and have difficulty breathing.

Guidelines: Caring for Clients with Angina Pectoris

G   Rest is extremely important. Rest reduces the heart's need for extra oxygen. It helps the blood flow return to normal, often within three to 15 minutes.

G   Medication is also needed to relax the walls of the coronary arteries. This allows them to open to get more blood to the heart. This medication, nitroglycerin, is a small tablet that the client places under the tongue. There it dissolves and is rapidly absorbed. Clients who have angina pectoris should keep nitroglycerin on hand to use as soon as symptoms arise. Home health aides are not allowed to give any medications. Tell your supervisor if the client needs help taking the medication. Nitroglycerin is also available as a patch. Do not remove the patch. Tell your supervisor immediately if the patch comes off. Nitroglycerin may also come in the form of a spray that the client sprays onto or under the tongue.

G Clients may also be required to avoid heavy meals, overeating, intense exercise, and cold, hot and humid weather.

Myocardial Infarction (MI) or Heart Attack

When blood flow to the heart muscle is completely blocked, oxygen and nutrients fail to reach the cells in that region. Waste products are not removed, and the muscle cell dies. This is called a myocardial infarction (MI), or heart attack. The area of dead tissue may be large or small, depending on the artery involved. Refer to the Medical Emergencies section for more information on signs and symptoms of MI.

Guidelines: Caring for Clients Recovering from Heart Attacks

G Most clients who have had an MI will be placed on a regular exercise program.

G Clients may be on a diet that is low in fat and cholesterol and/or a low-sodium diet.

G Medications may be prescribed to regulate heart rate and blood pressure.

G Quitting smoking will be encouraged.

G A stress management program may be started to help reduce stress levels.

G Clients may need to avoid cold temperatures.

Congestive Heart Failure (CHF)

Coronary artery disease, heart attack, hypertension, or other disorders may damage the heart. When the heart muscle has been severely damaged, it fails to pump effectively. Blood backs up into the heart instead of circulating. This is called **congestive heart failure**, or CHF. It can occur on one or both sides of the heart.

Guidelines: Caring for Clients with Congestive Heart Failure

G Medications can strengthen the heart muscle and improve its pumping.

G Medications help remove excess fluids. This means more trips to the bathroom. Assist clients as needed.

G A low-sodium diet or fluid restrictions may be prescribed.

G   A weakened heart may make it hard for clients to walk, carry items, or climb stairs. Limited activity or bedrest may be prescribed. Allow for a period of rest after an activity.

G   Intake of fluids and output of urine may need to be measured.

G   Client may weigh daily at the same time to note weight gain from fluid retention.

G   Elastic leg stockings may be applied to reduce swelling in feet and ankles.

G   Range of motion exercises improve muscle tone when activity and exercise are limited.

G   Extra pillows may help clients who have trouble breathing. Keeping the head of the bed elevated may also help with breathing.

G   Assistance with personal care and ADLs may need to be provided.

Report any of these to your supervisor:

G   Trouble breathing; coughing or gurgling with breathing

G   Dizziness, confusion, and fainting

G   Pale or blue skin

G   Low blood pressure

G   Swelling of the feet and ankles (edema)

G   Bulging veins in the neck

G   Weight gain

When a client has poor circulation to the legs and feet, elastic stockings are ordered. These stockings help prevent swelling and blood clots and improve circulation. These stockings are called "anti-embolic hose" or "elastic stockings." They need to be put on before the client gets out of bed. Follow manufacturer's instructions and illustrations for how to put on stockings.

Putting elastic stockings on a client

Equipment: elastic stockings

1. **Wash your hands.**

2. **Explain the procedure to the client, speaking clearly, slowly, and directly. Maintain face-to-face contact whenever possible.**

3. **Provide privacy for the client.**

4. **The client should be in the supine position (on his back) in bed. With client lying down, remove his or her socks, shoes, or slippers, and expose one leg.**

5. **Turn stocking inside out at least to heel area (Fig. 5-1).**

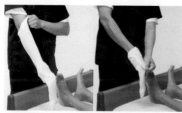

Fig. 5-1. Turning the stocking inside out allows stocking to roll on gently.

6. Gently place foot of stocking over toes, foot, and heel (Fig. 5-2). Make sure the heel is in the right place (heel should be in heel of stocking).

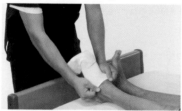

Fig. 5-2. Place the foot of the stocking over the toes, foot, and heel. Promote the client's comfort and safety. Avoid force and over-extension of joints.

7. Gently pull top of stocking over foot, heel, and leg.

8. Make sure there are no twists or wrinkles in stocking after it is on (Fig. 5-3). It must fit smoothly.

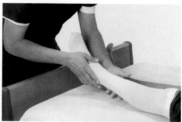

Fig. 5-3. Make stocking smooth. Twists or wrinkles cause the stocking to be too tight, which reduces circulation.

9. Repeat for other leg.

10. Wash your hands.

11. Document the procedure and your observations. How did the skin appear? Were there any changes in color or temperature? Were there any sores or swelling on the legs?

HIV and AIDS

Acquired immune deficiency syndrome (AIDS) is an illness caused by the human immunodeficiency virus (HIV). HIV attacks the body's immune system and gradually disables it. Eventually the person has weakened resistance to other infections. Death may be the result of these infections. However, medications can help people live longer. HIV is a sexually-transmitted disease. It is also spread through blood, infected needles, or to the fetus from its mother.

In general, HIV affects the body in stages. The first stage involves symptoms similar to flu, with fever, muscle aches, cough, and fatigue. These are signs of the immune system fighting the infection. As the infection worsens, the immune system overreacts. It attacks not only the virus, but also normal tissue.

When the virus weakens the immune system in later stages, a group of problems may appear. These include infections, tumors, and central nervous system symptoms. These problems would not occur if the immune system were healthy. This stage of the disease is known as AIDS.

In the late stages of AIDS, damage to the central nervous system may cause memory loss, poor coordination, paralysis, and confusion. These symptoms together are known as AIDS dementia complex.

The following are the signs and symptoms of HIV and AIDS:

- Appetite loss
- Involuntary weight loss of ten pounds or more
- Vague, flu-like symptoms, including fever, cough, weakness, and severe fatigue
- Night sweats
- Swollen lymph nodes in the neck, underarms, or groin
- Severe diarrhea
- Dry cough
- Skin rashes
- Painful white spots in the mouth or on the tongue
- Cold sores or fever blisters on the lips and flat, white ulcers in the mouth
- Cauliflower-like warts on the skin and in the mouth
- Inflamed and bleeding gums
- Low resistance to infection, particularly pneumonia, but also tuberculosis, herpes, bacterial infections, and hepatitis
- Bruising that does not go away
- Kaposi's sarcoma, a form of skin cancer that appears as purple or red skin lesions
- Pneumocystis pneumonia, a lung infection
- AIDS dementia complex

Infections, such as pneumonia, tuberculosis, or hepatitis, invade the body when the immune system is weak and cannot defend itself. These illnesses worsen AIDS. They further weaken the immune system. It is difficult to treat these infections. Over time, a person may develop a resistance to some antibiotics. These infections often cause death in people with AIDS.

Persons with HIV are treated with drugs that slow the progress of the disease, but do not cure it. The medicines must be taken at precise times. They have many unpleasant side effects. For some people, the medications work less well than for others. Other aspects of HIV treatment are relief of symptoms and prevention and treatment of infection. Follow Standard Precautions to help prevent the spread of HIV/AIDS.

You can provide valuable care for your clients who have HIV or AIDS. Their care will focus on the relief of symptoms and prevention of complications.

Guidelines: Caring for Clients with HIV/AIDS

G   People with poor immune system function are more sensitive to infections. Wash your hands often and keep everything clean.

G   Involuntary weight loss occurs in almost all people who develop AIDS. High-protein, high-calorie, and high-nutrient meals and supplements can help maintain a healthy weight.

G   Some people with HIV/AIDS lose their appetites and have trouble eating. Serve familiar and favorite foods in a pleasant setting. Report appetite loss or trouble eating to your supervisor.

G   Carefully follow guidelines for safe food preparation and storage when working with a client who has HIV/AIDS. Food-borne illnesses caused by improperly cooking or storing food can cause death for someone with HIV/AIDS. Wash your hands frequently. Keep everything clean, especially countertops, cutting boards, and knives after they have been used to cut meat. Thaw food in the refrigerator, and wash and cook foods thoroughly. When storing food, keep cold foods cold and hot foods hot. Use small containers that seal tightly. Check expiration dates, and remember, "when in doubt, throw it out."

G   Clients who have infections of the mouth and esophagus may need food that is low in acid and neither cold nor hot. Spicy seasonings should not be used. Soft or pureed foods may be easier to swallow. Liquid meals and fortified drinks, such as milk shakes, may ease the pain of chewing. Warm salt water or other rinses may help painful sores of the mouth. Good mouth care is essential.

G   A person who has nausea or vomiting should eat small, frequent meals, if possible. The person should eat slowly. The person should avoid high-fat and spicy foods, and eat a soft, bland diet. This includes mashed potatoes, noodles, rice, crackers, pretzels, toast, gelatin, and clear soups. Cold foods that have little odor are usually easier to eat than hot foods. When nausea and vomiting persist, liquids and salty foods should be encouraged. These include clear soups, clear juices, ginger ale and colas, saltines, and pretzels. Clients should eat small, frequent meals and drink fluids in between meals. Care must be taken to maintain proper intake of fluids to balance lost fluids.

G   Clients who have mild diarrhea may have frequent small meals that are low in fat, fiber, and milk products. If diarrhea is severe, the doctor may order a "BRAT" diet (a diet of bananas, rice, apples, and toast). This diet is helpful for short-term use. Diarrhea rapidly depletes the body of fluids. Fluid replacement is necessary. Good rehydration fluids include water, juice, soda, and broth. Caffeinated drinks should be avoided.

G   **Neuropathy**, or numbness, tingling, and pain in the feet and legs is usually treated with medications. Going without shoes or wearing loose, soft slippers may help. If blankets cause pain, use a bed cradle to keep sheets and blankets from resting on the legs and feet.

G   Clients with HIV/AIDS may suffer from anxiety and depression. They often suffer the judgments of family, friends, and society. Some people blame them for their illness. People with HIV/AIDS may have tremendous stress. They may feel uncertainty about their illness, health care, and finances. They may also have lost people in their social support network of friends and family. Clients with this disease need support from others. This may come from family, friends, religious and community groups, and support groups, as well as the care team. Treat all your clients with respect and help provide the emotional support they need.

G   Withdrawal, avoidance of tasks, and mental slowness are early symptoms of HIV. Medications may also cause side effects of this type. Later, AIDS dementia complex may cause further mental symptoms. There may also be muscle weakness and loss of muscle control, making falls a risk. Clients will need a safe environment and close supervision in their ADLs.

Dementia

As we age, we may lose some of our ability to think logically and quickly. This ability is called cognition. Loss of this ability is called cognitive impairment. Cognitive impairment affects concentration and memory. Elderly clients may lose their memories of recent events, which can be frustrating for them. You can help. Encourage them to make lists of things to remember. Write down names, events, and phone numbers. Other normal changes of aging in the brain include slower reaction time, trouble finding or using the right words, and sleeping less.

Dementia is a general term that refers to a serious loss of mental abilities such as thinking, remembering, reasoning, and communicating. As dementia advances, these losses make it difficult to perform ADLs such as eating, bathing, dressing, and toileting. Dementia is not a normal part of aging.

The following are some causes of dementia:

- Alzheimer's disease
- Multi-infarct dementia or vascular dementia (a series of strokes that damage the brain)
- Lewy body dementia
- Parkinson's disease
- Huntington's disease

Alzheimer's Disease (AD)

Alzheimer's disease (AD) causes tangled nerve fibers and protein deposits to form in the brain, eventually causing dementia. The disease gets worse, causing greater and greater loss of health and abilities. There is no known cause of Alzheimer's disease and there is no cure. Clients with Alzheimer's disease will never recover. They will need more care as the disease progresses.

Alzheimer's disease generally begins with forgetfulness and confusion. It progresses to complete loss of all ability to care for oneself. Each person with AD will show different symptoms at different times. For example, one person with AD may be able to read, but may not be able to use the phone or remember her own address. Another person may have lost the ability to read, but may still be able to do simple math. Skills a person has used constantly over a long lifetime are usually kept longer.

Encourage clients with Alzheimer's disease to perform ADLs. Help them keep their minds and bodies as active as possible. Working, socializing, reading, problem solving, and exercising should all be encouraged. Having them do as much as possible for themselves may even help slow the progression of the disease. Look for tasks that are challenging but not frustrating. Help your clients succeed in doing them.

These attitudes will help you give the best possible care to your clients with Alzheimer's disease:

- Do not take their behavior personally.
- Put yourself in their shoes.
- Treat clients with Alzheimer's disease with dignity and respect, as you would want to be treated.

- Work with the symptoms and behaviors you see.
- Work as a team.
- Encourage communication.
- Take care of yourself.
- Work with family members.
- Remember the goals of the care plan.

Guidelines: Communicating with Clients Who Have Alzheimer's Disease

G Always approach from the front. Do not startle the client.

G Determine how close the client wants you to be.

G Speak in a low, calm voice, in a room with little background noise and distraction.

G Use the client's name during the conversation.

G Speak slower, using a lower tone of voice than normal.

G Repeat yourself, using the same words and phrases as often as needed.

G Use signs, pictures, gestures, or written words to help communicate.

G Break complex tasks into smaller, simpler ones.

Use the same procedures for personal care and ADLs for clients with Alzheimer's disease as you would with other clients. However, there are some guidelines to keep in mind when helping these clients. These general principles will help you give the best care:

1. Develop a routine and stick to it. Being consistent is very important for clients who are confused and easily upset.

2. Promote self-care. Help your clients to care for themselves as much as possible. This will help them cope with this difficult disease.

3. Take good care of yourself, both mentally and physically. This will help you give the best care.

Guidelines: Caring for Clients with Alzheimer's Disease

G Encourage fluids. Never withhold or discourage fluids because a person is incontinent. Follow schedules for toileting.

G Mark the bathroom with a sign as a reminder of where it is and to use the toilet.

G Put lids on trash cans, waste baskets, or other containers if the client has a habit of urinating in them.

G   Lay out clothes in the order in which they should be put on. Choose clothes that are simple to put on.

G   Schedule bathing when the client is least agitated. Be organized so the bath can be quick.

G   Be flexible about bathing. Your client may not always be in the mood. Be relaxed. Allow the client to enjoy the bath. Check the skin regularly when bathing for signs of irritation.

G   Ensure safety by using non-slip mats, tub seats, and hand-holds.

G   Maintain proper nutrition. Schedule meals at the same time each day. Serve familiar foods. Try smaller, more frequent meals if person is restless. Finger foods can allow eating while moving around. Keep bite-sized snacks nearby, especially favorites.

G   Do not serve steaming or very hot foods or drinks. Use dishes without a pattern. White usually works best. Put only one item of food on the plate at a time.

G   Guide the client through meals. Provide simple instructions. Offer regular drinks of water, juice, and other fluids to avoid dehydration.

G   Assist with grooming. Help the people in your care feel attractive and dignified.

G   Prevent infections. Follow proper procedures for food preparation and storage, household management, and Standard Precautions.

G   Maintain a daily exercise routine.

G   Maintain self-esteem by encouraging independence in ADLs.

G   Share in enjoyable activities, looking at pictures, talking, and reminiscing.

G   Reward positive and independent behavior with smiles, hugs, warm touches, and thanks.

Below are some common difficult behaviors that you may face when working with Alzheimer's clients:

Agitation: Try to eliminate triggers. Keep routine constant. Avoid frustration. Help client focus on a soothing, familiar activity, such as sorting things or looking at pictures. Remain calm. Use a low, soothing voice to speak to and reassure the client. An arm around the shoulder, patting, or stroking may be soothing for some clients.

Sundowning: When a person becomes restless and agitated in the late afternoon, evening, or night, it is called **sundowning**. Remove triggers. Provide snacks or encourage rest. Avoid stressful situations during this time. Limit activities, appointments, trips, and visits. Play soft music. Set a bedtime routine and keep it. Recognize when sundowning occurs and plan a calming activity just before. Remove caffeine from the diet. Give a soothing back massage. Distract the client with a simple, calm activity like looking at a magazine. Maintain a daily exercise routine.

Violent Behavior: A client who attacks, hits, or threatens someone is violent. Frustration, overstimulation, or a change in routine, environment, or caregiver may trigger violence. Look for ways to avoid these triggers. These are appropriate responses to violent clients:

- Block blows, but never hit back.
- Step out of reach.
- Call for help if needed.
- Do not leave client in the home alone.
- Try to eliminate triggers.
- Use techniques to calm client as you would for agitation or sundowning.

Pacing and Wandering: A client who walks back and forth in the same area is pacing. A client who walks aimlessly around the house or neighborhood is wandering. Pacing and wandering may be caused by restlessness, hunger, disorientation, need for toileting, constipation, pain, forgetting how or where to sit down, too much daytime napping, or the need for exercise. Remove causes when you can. For example, give nutritious snacks and maintain a toileting schedule. Let clients pace and wander in a safe and secure (locked) area where you can watch them. Suggest another activity, such as going for a walk together.

Hallucinations or Delusions: A client who sees, hears, smells, tastes, or feels things that are not there is having hallucinations. A client who believes things that are not true is having delusions. Ignore harmless hallucinations and delusions. Reassure a client who seems agitated or worried. Do not argue with a client who is imagining things. Do not tell the client that you can see or hear his or her hallucinations. Redirect the client to other activities or thoughts. Be calm and reassure client that you are there to help.

Depression: Report signs of depression to your supervisor immediately. It is an illness that can be treated with medication. Encourage independence, self-care, and activity. Talk about moods and feelings if the client wishes. Be a good listener. Encourage social interaction.

Perseveration or Repetitive Phrasing: A client who repeats a word, phrase, question, or activity over and over is **perseverating**. Respond to perseveration with patience. Do not try to silence or stop the client. Answer questions each time they are asked, using the same words each time.

Disruptiveness: Disruptive behavior is anything that disturbs others, such as yelling, banging on furniture, slamming doors, etc. Often this behavior is triggered by a wish for attention, by pain or constipation, or by frustration. When this behavior happens, gain the client's attention. Be calm and friendly. Try to find out why the behavior is happening. To try to prevent this behavior, notice and praise improvements in the client's behavior. Be tactful and sensitive when you do this. Do not treat the client like a child. Tell the client about any changes in schedules, routines, or the environment in advance. Involve the client in developing routine activities and schedules. Encourage the client to join in independent activities that are safe (for example, folding towels). This can prevent feelings of powerlessness. Help the client find ways to cope. Focus on positive activities he or she may still be able to do, such as knitting, crocheting, crafts, etc.

Inappropriate Social Behavior: Inappropriate social behavior may be cursing, name calling, or other behavior. As with violent or disruptive behavior, there may be many reasons why a client is behaving this way. Try not to take it personally. The client may only be reacting to frustration or other stress, not to you. Stay calm. Be reassuring. Try to find out what caused the behavior (for example, too much noise, too many people, too much stress, pain, or discomfort). Respond positively to any appropriate behavior. Report any physical abuse or serious verbal abuse to your supervisor.

Inappropriate Sexual Behavior: Inappropriate sexual behavior, such as removing clothes, touching one's own genitals, or trying to touch others can embarrass those who see it. Be matter-of-fact when dealing with such behavior. Do not overreact. This may reinforce the behavior. Be sensitive to the nature of the problem. Try to distract the client. A client may be reacting to a need for physical stimulation or affection. Consider other ways to provide physical stimulation. Try backrubs, a soft doll or stuffed animal to cuddle, comforting blankets, or pieces of cloth.

Although Alzheimer's disease cannot be cured, there are techniques that can improve the quality of life for clients with AD.

Reality orientation involves the use of calendars, clocks, signs, and lists to help clients remember who and where they are. It is useful in the early stages of Alzheimer's disease when clients are confused but not totally disoriented. In later stages, reality orientation may only frustrate clients.

Validation therapy is letting clients believe they live in the past or in imaginary circumstances. **Validating** means giving value to or approving. Make no attempt to reorient clients to actual circumstances. Explore clients' beliefs. Do not argue with them. It is useful in cases of moderate to severe disorientation.

Reminiscence therapy is encouraging clients to remember and talk about the past. Explore memories by asking about details. Focus on a time of life that was more pleasant. Work through feelings about a difficult time in the past. It is useful in many stages of Alzheimer's disease, but especially with moderate to severe confusion.

Activity therapy uses activities clients enjoy to prevent boredom and frustration. These activities also promote self-esteem. Help clients to take walks, do puzzles, listen to music, cook, read, or do other activities they enjoy. It is useful throughout most stages of Alzheimer's disease.

Chronic Obstructive Pulmonary Disease (COPD)

Chronic obstructive pulmonary disease, or COPD, is a chronic disease. This means the client may live for years with it but never be cured. Clients with COPD have difficulty breathing, especially in getting air out of the lungs. There are two chronic lung diseases that are grouped under COPD: chronic bronchitis and emphysema.

Over time, a client with either of these lung disorders becomes chronically ill and weakened. There is a high risk for acute lung infections, such as pneumonia. When the lungs and brain do not get enough oxygen, all body systems are affected. Clients may live with a constant fear of not being able to breathe. This can cause them to sit upright in an attempt to improve their ability to expand the lungs. These clients can have poor appetites. They usually do not get enough sleep. All of this can add to their feelings of weakness and poor health. They may feel they have lost control of their bodies, particularly with breathing. They may fear suffocation.

Clients with COPD may experience the following symptoms:

- Chronic cough or wheeze
- Trouble breathing, especially with inhaling and exhaling deeply
- Shortness of breath, especially during physical exertion
- Pale or cyanotic (blue) skin or reddish-purple skin

- Confusion
- General state of weakness
- Trouble completing meals due to shortness of breath
- Fear and anxiety

Guidelines: Caring for Clients with COPD

G Colds or viruses can quickly make clients very ill. Always observe and report signs of symptoms getting worse.

G Help clients sit upright or lean forward. Offer pillows to support them.

G Offer plenty of fluids and small, frequent meals.

G Encourage a well-balanced diet.

G Keep oxygen supply available as ordered.

G Being unable to breathe or fearing suffocation can be very frightening. Be calm and supportive.

G Use good infection control, especially with handwashing by the client and the disposal of used tissues.

G Encourage as much independence with ADLs as possible.

G Remind clients to avoid situations where they may be exposed to infections, especially colds and the flu.

G Encourage pursed-lip breathing. Pursed-lip breathing is placing the lips as if in a kiss and taking controlled breaths.

G Encourage clients to save energy for important tasks. Encourage clients to rest.

Tuberculosis (TB)

Tuberculosis, or TB, is an airborne disease carried on mucous droplets suspended in the air. When a person infected with TB talks, coughs, breathes, or sings, he may release mucous droplets carrying the disease. TB usually infects the lungs, causing coughing, difficulty breathing, fever, and fatigue. It can be cured. However, if left untreated, TB may cause death.

Symptoms of TB include fatigue, loss of appetite, weight loss, slight fever and chills, night sweats, prolonged coughing, coughing up blood, chest pain, shortness of breath, and trouble breathing.

When caring for clients who have TB, follow Standard Precautions and

Airborne Precautions. Wear a mask and gown during client care. Use special care when handling sputum. Follow isolation procedures if directed. Help the client remember to take all medication prescribed. Failure to do so is a major factor in the spread of TB. Multidrug-resistant TB (MDR TB) can develop when people with TB disease do not take all the prescribed medication.

Hip/Knee Replacement

Total hip replacement is surgery that replaces the head of the long bone of the leg (femur) where it joins the hip. This may be done for any of these reasons:

- Fractured hip due to an injury or fall which does not heal properly
- Weakened hip due to aging
- Hip causes extreme pain and disability because the joint is badly damaged from osteoarthritic changes. The bones are no longer strong enough to bear the person's weight.

After the surgery, the client cannot stand on that leg while the area heals. A physical therapist will play an important role after surgery. The goals of care include slowly strengthening the hip muscles and getting the client walking on that leg. Be familiar with the care plan. It will state when the client may begin to put weight on the leg. It will also tell how much the client is able to do. Help with personal care and with using assistive devices, such as walkers or canes.

Guidelines: Caring for Clients Recovering from Hip Replacements

G Keep often-used items, such as telephone, tissues, call signals, and water within easy reach. Avoid placing items in high places.

G Dress starting with the affected (weaker) side first.

G Never rush the client. Use praise and encouragement often. Do this even for small accomplishments.

G Have the client sit to do tasks to save his or her energy.

G Follow the care plan exactly, even if the client wants to do more than is ordered.

G Never perform range of motion exercises on a leg on the side of a hip replacement unless directed by your supervisor.

G Caution the client not to cross legs or turn toes inward. The hip cannot be bent or flexed more than 90 degrees. The hip cannot be turned inward or outward.

G   When transferring from the bed, stand on the side of the unaffected hip so that the strong side leads in standing, pivoting, and sitting. With chair or toilet transfers, the stronger leg should stand first.

G   Report any of the following to your supervisor:

- Redness, drainage, bleeding, or warmth in incision area
- An increase in pain
- Numbness or tingling
- Abnormal vital signs, especially change in temperature
- Client cannot use equipment properly and safely
- Client is not following doctor's orders for activity and exercise
- Any problems with appetite
- Any improvements, such as increased strength and improved ability to walk

Knee replacement is the surgical insertion of a prosthetic knee. A **prosthesis** is a device that replaces a body part that is missing or deformed because of an accident, injury, illness, or birth defect. It is used to improve a person's ability to function and/or his appearance. Knee replacement surgery is performed to relieve pain. It also restores motion to a knee damaged by injury or arthritis. It can help stabilize a knee that buckles or gives out repeatedly. Care is similar to that for the hip replacement, but the recovery time is much shorter. These clients have more ability to care for themselves. Therefore, they are not seen in home care as often as clients with hip replacements.

Guidelines: Knee Replacement

G   To prevent blood clots, apply special stockings as ordered.

G   Perform ankle pumps as ordered. These are simple exercises that promote circulation to the legs. Ankle pumps are done by raising the toes and feet toward the ceiling and lowering them again.

G   Encourage fluids, especially cranberry and orange juice, which contain Vitamin C, to prevent urinary tract infections (UTIs).

G   Assist with deep breathing exercises as ordered.

G   Report to your supervisor if you notice redness, swelling, heat, or deep tenderness in one or both calves.

VI.
Home Management and Nutrition

The Client's Environment

Housekeeping

Providing a safe, clean, and orderly environment has always been an essential part of home health care. Clients feel better physically and psychologically and recover more quickly when their homes and families receive care and support. Infection and accidents are prevented. You will be a role model for your clients and their families.

It takes efficiency, planning, knowledge, and skills to manage a household. You will need to know how to use your time and energy well. This is so that you do not neglect your primary responsibility—the personal care of the client. Sensitivity is another important quality when caring for your clients' homes. You must respect the customs, beliefs, and feelings of your clients and their families.

Your assignments will vary. They may include simple cleaning and organizing of the client's room or general cleaning throughout the house. Some clients require management of all household functions, including finances. You may be required to dust, straighten up, vacuum, sweep, wash dishes, clean the bathroom and kitchen, and do laundry. Your assignments will outline the specific duties to be performed. Most agencies require that HHAs perform light housekeeping. This usually involves dusting, straightening, vacuuming or sweeping floors, cleaning bathrooms and the kitchen, and disposing of trash.

Guidelines: Housekeeping

G   Invite family participation. Depending on their abilities and availability, clients and family members may be asked to participate in housekeeping tasks.

G   Invite family and client input when you determine the tasks that need to be done and the methods used.

G   Use cleaning materials and methods that are acceptable to and approved by clients and their families.

G   Any efforts you make toward improving the home environment should coincide with the client's choices, lifestyle, and values.

G   Be organized when performing tasks. Write out detailed daily and weekly schedules. Seek feedback from your supervisor and the client and family.

G   Build some flexibility in the schedule to allow for changes in the client's condition, needs, appointments, or social activities.

G   Organize cleaning materials and equipment by placing them in one closet. Do not leave cleaning equipment around the home.

G   Familiarize yourself with the household's cleaning materials and equipment. Read the labels and instruction booklets.

G   Maintain a safe environment, as well as a clean and healthy one. Do not wax floors if your client is unsteady. Mop up spills immediately.

G   Use housekeeping procedures and methods that promote good health.

G   Observe the home for signs of infestation by roaches, rats, mice, lice, and fleas. Report to your supervisor if you note signs of infestation.

G   Use good body mechanics while performing home maintenance activities to prevent injury.

G   Clean up and straighten up after every activity. Spills that have dried are difficult to remove later.

G   Carry paper and a small pencil to make note of items that must be purchased or replaced. Maintain a shopping list on a bulletin board, refrigerator door, or other convenient location. Encourage family members to use the list.

G   Use your time wisely and efficiently. For example, prepare food while a load of wash is being done.

All cleaning products must be used properly. With the exception of some non-toxic types, cleaning products are chemicals, which can be irritating and can even cause burns. Some chemicals are poisonous when swallowed.

Guidelines: Using Household Cleaning Products

G   Read and follow the directions on the label of every product you use. Cleaning products can harm the materials and surfaces you are trying to clean.

G   Do not mix cleaning products. The fumes are toxic and can be fatal.

G   Open windows when cleaning to provide fresh air. Some cleaning products may have fumes that are unpleasant or even harmful if you are exposed to them for a long time.

G   Do not leave cleaning products on surfaces longer than the recommended time. Do not scrub too hard on some surfaces.

Not all housekeeping tasks must be performed daily. Some tasks may be done weekly. Others only need to be done once a month or seasonally. Space out the special tasks. Do each cleaning job properly and efficiently. Do not take a lot of steps and do not reach, bend, and stoop unnecessarily. Experiment a little to find the most comfortable and effective way to do a job. Cleaning can be done when your client is resting, sleeping, or doing another activity. Care of the client is your primary responsibility. However, do not neglect housekeeping.

Guidelines: Straightening and Cleaning Living Areas

G   Clear up clutter and put objects in their correct places.

G   Pick up newspapers, magazines, and toys as needed.

G   Empty wastebaskets and ashtrays daily.

G   Make the beds each day.

G   Keep essential and frequently-used items, such as eyeglasses, tissues, wastebaskets, newspapers, magazines, and books, within reach.

G   Dust once a week or when necessary. If your client has allergies, you may need to dust daily.

G   Vacuum floors and rugs once a week or more often if indicated. If the home does not have a vacuum, use a broom to sweep the floors and rugs. Take care not to raise much dust.

G   Floors covered with vinyl, ceramic tile, and linoleum may be washed. Some wood floors may not. Check with the client or family members before you begin. After removing loose dirt or crumbs with a vacuum or broom, wash floors with a cloth or mop dipped in warm sudsy water. Dry the floor after you have washed it or close off the area for the time it takes for the floor to dry.

Handling food on contaminated surfaces, improper dishwashing, and contaminated food storage areas may transmit many diseases. Roaches, rats, and mice may cause disease and allergy by contaminating food with their saliva or through their droppings. Pest control is vital to health and cleanliness. Always report pest control problems to your supervisor.

Guidelines: Cleaning the Kitchen

G Clean the kitchen after every use. Ask family members to do the same. Do not wait until the end of the day to clean up. Daily kitchen cleaning tasks include washing dishes, wiping surfaces, taking out garbage, and storing leftover food. Weekly tasks include cleaning the refrigerator and washing the floor. Cleaning cabinets, drawers, and other storage areas is usually done a few times a year.

G Wash dishes in hot soapy water using liquid dish detergent. Rinse them in hot water. When working with clients who have an infectious disease or a cold, use boiling water for rinsing and add a tablespoon of chlorine bleach to the soapy water. The combination of heat and chlorine will kill pathogens, or harmful microorganisms.

G Wash glasses and cups first, then silverware, plates, and bowls. Pots and pans are washed last. Rinse with hot water and dry on a rack. Air drying dishes is more sanitary than drying with a dish towel.

G If the house has a dishwasher, learn how to correctly load and start it. Dishwashers save time. They may also sterilize dishes due to the high temperatures used in washing and drying.

G Do not wash the following items in the dishwasher: electrical appliances, certain plastic materials, wooden pieces or utensils, hand-painted or antique dishes, delicate china, crystal, cast iron, most pots and pans, and sharp or carbon steel knives.

G Use only a dishwasher detergent in the dishwasher. Fill the well with only the amount recommended on the label.

G The refrigerator should be totally cleaned once a week. However, you should wipe it out more frequently. If the refrigerator is not a self-defrosting one, the freezer should be defrosted whenever necessary. To defrost a freezer, turn the dial to the "off" position. Read the directions on the freezer.

G Mix two tablespoons of baking soda in one quart of warm water. Wipe the inside walls of the refrigerator and freezer. Baking soda will remove odors. Wash the shelves and trays with warm, soapy water.

G Clean countertops, tables, and the stove each time they are used. Clean the outside of the stove, the trays, and burners with hot, sudsy water or an all-purpose cleaner, and rinse. Ovens should be cleaned according to manufacturer's recommendations. Be sure to follow the directions. Clean cabinet and drawer fronts once a week. If a cutting board or other surface has been used to cut fresh meat, scrub the surface thoroughly with soapy water. Rinse well.

G An all-purpose cleaner may be needed to remove grease and cooked foods that have spilled or splashed on surfaces. Clean the sink with a cleanser such as scouring powder or cream.

G Never place food on soiled work or storage areas or in unclean containers. Keep food covered. Close lids of cartons and cover food storage containers to prevent contamination or infestation by insects and rodents. Place leftovers in covered containers and store them in the refrigerator immediately. Use them within two to three days.

G Vacuum, sweep, or dry mop the floor daily. Damp mop uncarpeted floors at least once a week, using hot water and a floor cleaner. Rinse the floor if label recommends doing so. Dry the floor or close off the area until the floor dries to prevent accidents.

G Dispose of garbage daily. To prevent odor and discourage insects and rodents, rinse out tin cans and bottles before placing them in the garbage pail or recycling bin. Follow the recycling procedures for your client's community. Periodically wash wastebaskets and trash cans with hot, soapy water.

G Store all cleaning materials away from food, food preparation utensils, and food preparation areas. Keep them out of reach of children and confused clients.

A clean, organized, and odor-free bathroom is an important part of improving a family's hygiene and safety. Because it is moist and warm, the bathroom is a reservoir for the growth of microorganisms, mold, and mildew.

Guidelines: Cleaning the Bathroom

G Involve the entire family in keeping the bathroom clean. Always wash from clean areas to dirty areas, so you do not spread dirt into areas that have already been washed.

G Flush the toilet each time it is used.

G Clean toothbrushes and toothbrush holders.

G Scrub the tub and shower after use.

G Remove hair from drain strainers.

G Hang up all used towels to dry.

G   Put away toiletries.

G   Rinse the sink after brushing teeth, shaving, and washing.

G   Place soiled towels in the laundry hamper after they are dry.

The bathroom is the location of many home accidents. Make sure that all bathroom rugs are non-skid. Wipe up puddles of water immediately. If grab bars are not present and your client has difficulty moving about in the bathroom safely, report this to your supervisor.

Cleaning the bathroom

Equipment: approved disinfectant (a cleaning product that kills germs), scouring powder or scouring cream with bleach, sponges, toilet brush, glass cleaner, paper towels, disposable or rubber gloves

1. **Put on gloves.**

2. **Using the disinfectant and sponge (or paper towels), wipe all surfaces and rinse as needed. Be sure to clean the sides, walls, and curtain or door of the shower or tub; the towel racks; holders for toilet paper, toothbrushes, and soap; and window sills.**

3. **Rinse sponge well. Use a different sponge to wipe the outside of the toilet bowl, seat, and lid. As a general cleaning rule, start with the cleanest surface first, then move to dirtier areas.**

4. **Use a different sponge to clean the bathtub, shower stall, and sink. Use scouring powder or cream for tile and porcelain, and disinfectant or all-purpose cleaner on other surfaces. Remember that scouring powder can scratch. Check with the client or a family member before using it. Be sure to scrub the sides, edges, and bottoms of all these areas. Clean faucets and scrub around their bases.**

5. **Scrub the inside of the toilet bowl with a brush and scouring powder containing bleach. Be sure to scrub under the rim. If you use a second, stronger toilet cleaner, flush the first cleaning product down the drain first to avoid possible chemical reactions. Wash the toilet brush with a disinfectant solution. Store it in a holder or plastic bag after letting it air dry.**

6. **Vacuum or dry mop the floor first, then wash if the floor is tile or linoleum. Use an all-purpose floor cleaner in hot water. Wash the floor with a cloth or mop, taking special care to clean the areas at the base of the toilet and sink. Do not leave the floor wet. Dry it carefully to avoid accidents.**

7. **Clean the mirror and any glass or chrome surfaces using glass cleaner and paper towels or clean rags.**

8. **Place dry, soiled towels in the laundry hamper. Empty the waste can into a plastic or paper garbage bag and dispose of it. Replace toilet tissue and facial tissue when needed. Open the bathroom window for a short time, if possible, to air the room out. Once a week, wash out the waste can and**

laundry hamper, and launder the bath mats and rugs.

9. Store supplies.

10. Remove and discard gloves.

11. Wash your hands.

12. Document the cleaning.

Guidelines: Cleaning and Organizing Storage Areas

G Every item in the home should have a storage place that is convenient for use. That means storage places should be as close as possible to where items are used. For example, bath towels should be stored in or near the bathroom. Items that are used together should be stored near each other. Arrange food on shelves according to category. Store dangerous materials out of reach of children and confused adults.

G Some storage areas only need to be cleaned occasionally. Remove the stored items. Wipe the shelves and drawers with a damp cloth and cleaner. Clean food storage areas more often.

G Do not change the client's or the family's storage arrangements without talking to them. If you think changes are needed, discuss your ideas with the family.

Cleaning Solution Ideas

Several types of cleaning solutions can be prepared from common household items when supplies are not available or when the family budget is restricted. Some of these are environmentally safe and non-toxic.

- Baking soda can be used instead of scouring powder. Baking soda can also be diluted with warm water to make a solution that will eliminate odors when used to clean surfaces.

- White vinegar can be used to remove lime or other mineral deposits on sinks, toilets, or chrome fixtures. White vinegar diluted with water can be used instead of glass cleaner. Mix solution using one part white vinegar to three parts water (1:3).

- Household bleach, diluted with four parts water, makes a strong disinfectant solution to clean bathroom surfaces. Diluted with nine parts water and stored in a spray or pour bottle, bleach makes a milder disinfectant to use on kitchen counters.

Most house-cleaning tasks should be done either immediately, daily, weekly, monthly, or less often. Take into account the care plan, your assigned tasks, how much help is needed, and how much time you have in a particular home to prepare a cleaning schedule. You may not always stick to the schedule exactly. However, it will guide your work and help you get essential cleaning done. Establishing a schedule for cleaning can also help the family keep a housekeeping routine after your care has ended.

You must follow Standard Precautions with every client. This is true because you cannot know when infection is present. However, when a client has a known infectious disease, such as influenza, or one that weakens the immune system, such as AIDS or cancer, you need to take special precautions in housecleaning:

- Use disinfectant when cleaning countertops and surfaces in the kitchen and bathroom.

- Clean the client's bathroom daily. Have other family members use a different bathroom if possible.

- Use separate dishes and utensils for the infected client. In some cases, disposable dishes and utensils will be ordered.

- Wash dishes and utensils in the dishwasher or wash dishes in hot soapy water with bleach. Rinse in boiling water, and allow to air dry.

- Disinfect any surfaces that contact body fluids, such as bedpans, urinals and toilets.

- Frequently remove trash containing used tissues.

- Keep any specimens of urine, stool, or sputum in double bags and away from food and food preparation areas.

Laundry

You may be expected to do hand or machine washing as part of an assignment. Clean clothes, bed linens, and towels are important for hygiene and comfort.

Laundry Products and Equipment: To do the laundry you will need laundry detergent, a washing machine or a basin for hand washing clothes, and a dryer or a clothesline and clothespins. The instructions for using washing machines are usually located on the inside of the washing machine lid. In general, you will use all-purpose detergent. Energy-efficient washing machines usually require a high-efficiency (HE) laundry detergent. Some delicate fabrics, underwear, or stockings may require a special detergent. Some clients may prefer a non-detergent soap for use on baby clothes and diapers. Bleach, color brighteners, stain removers, and fabric softeners may also be used. Ask the client and family members about their preferences for laundry products.

Pretreating: Pretreating means giving special treatment to items that have heavy soil, spots, and stains before washing them. Spots and stains should be treated immediately. The sooner they are treated, the easier they are to remove. Some oily stains harden with age and cannot be removed.

Bleach: Bleach is used with detergent. However, bleach cannot be used on all fabrics. Be familiar with the type of bleach and the fabric that is being washed. Three types of bleach are used in laundry: liquid chlorine, powdered chlorine, and oxygen or all-fabric. Each type of bleach should be used with caution. Read the instructions on the container carefully before using it.

Water Temperature: Read the washing instructions for all materials and garments. Warm water is the safest temperature for most garments. However, some must be washed in cold to prevent shrinking or colors fading. Hot water is generally used for towels, bed linens, and white or colorfast cottons. Warm is usually used for permanent press, knit, synthetic, sheer, lace, acetate, fabric blends, washable rayons, and plastic. Cold water is used for brightly-colored fabrics or fabrics that are not colorfast.

Washing Action or Cycle: Use the normal setting on the washer for cottons, linens, rayons, sturdy permanent press, knits, synthetics, blends, and most other items. Set the washer on the slow or gentle setting for washable woolens, old quilts, curtains, and delicate or fragile items.

Drying Clothes: Settings on the dryer vary according to the model. Most dryers have a permanent press setting and a delicate setting. The more delicate a fabric, the lower the drying temperature and the shorter the time in the dryer. Heavy items such as towels need higher temperature settings and a longer time in the dryer. Clean the lint filter each time you use the dryer. If your client does not have a clothes dryer, hang clothes on a clothesline using clothespins.

Folding: To reduce the amount of wrinkling, remove all clothes from the dryer immediately. Fold them neatly or place them on hangers. Set aside those that need to be ironed. Return other items to their drawers.

Ironing: Before you begin to iron, check the label of the item for the recommended temperature. If the label does not recommend a particular setting or the fabric is a blend, use the lowest temperature on the iron. Take special care with pile fabrics, such as velvets and corduroy. They will keep their texture better if ironed on the wrong side, with the iron placed over a towel. Dark fabrics, silks, acetates, rayons, linens, and some wools must be pressed on the wrong side to prevent them from becoming shiny. Use a pressing cloth to protect the fabric.

Maintaining Clothing: You may need to do basic mending or sewing occasionally. This is especially true if you are taking care of a family, an older person with impaired vision, or people who may not have the time or the ability to keep clothing and linens repaired. Some clients who can do their own mending may just need you to thread the needle.

Doing the laundry

1. **Sort clothes carefully. Make separate piles of whites, colors, and bright colors. Check clothing labels for special washing instructions. Do not wash anything labeled "Dry Clean Only." If hand washing is recommended, do not wash in the machine.**

2. **As you sort laundry, check pockets and remove tissues, money, pens, and other items. Remove belts with buckles, trims, and non-washable ornaments. Close zippers, buttons, and other fasteners. Check garments for stains and areas of heavy soil. If appropriate, mend or repair any holes, snags, rips, tears, pulled seams, and weak spots in garments and other items.**

3. **Pretreat spots and stains before washing (Fig. 6-1). A small amount of liquid detergent or dry detergent dissolved in water can be worked in with an old toothbrush. Pretreat or soak clothing as soon as possible for best results. If you know something is spotted, do not let it sit in the laundry hamper all week until you do the laundry.**

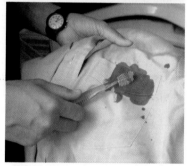

Fig. 6-1. Pretreating helps remove spots, stains, and areas that are heavily soiled.

4. **Use the correct water temperature: hot for whites, warm for colors, cold for bright colors.**

5. **Use the appropriate laundry product(s). Follow the washing instructions on the container.**

6. **Follow written instructions or client or family instructions for using the washer. Use the correct washing cycle for the load you are laundering.**

7. **Dry clothes completely, either in a dryer or on a clothesline. If using a dryer, follow the drying instructions on clothing labels or the client's preferences. Some fabrics require cooler temperatures.**

8. **Hand-wash items in warm or cool water, depending on the fabric and instructions. Use a mild detergent or special hand-washing liquid. Line dry or lay items flat on towels to preserve the shape of the garment.**

9. **Fold or hang clean laundry and sort into categories. Store in drawers or closets.**

When a client has a known infectious disease, you must take special precautions when handling laundry:

- Keep client's laundry separate from that of other family members.
- Handle dirty laundry as little as possible. Do not shake it. Sort it and put it in plastic bags in the client's room or bathroom. Take it immediately to the laundry area. Keep laundry off the floor.
- Wear gloves and hold laundry away from your clothes and body when you are handling it.
- Use liquid bleach when fabrics allow.
- Use agency-approved disinfectants in all loads.
- Use hot water.

In some assignments, you will be asked to teach housekeeping skills to family members. This prepares them to take over housekeeping and care when home care is discontinued. By teaching household management skills, you help families meet their daily needs and become more self-reliant.

Guidelines: Teaching Family Members

G   Get to know the family before starting to teach them. Understand their needs or problems before beginning.

G   Be patient. Give people time to learn new skills. Praise their efforts.

G   Keep teaching sessions brief.

G   Break down tasks into simple steps. Explain each step and demonstrate it.

G   Answer all questions.

G   Assist the person as necessary. Do not do the task for him or her.

G   Remember that each person is an individual and will learn in different ways. Customize your teaching to allow for these differences.

Bedmaking

Some clients spend much or all of their time in bed. Careful bedmaking is essential to their comfort, cleanliness, and health. Linens should always be changed after personal care procedures such as sponge baths, or any time bedding or sheets are damp, soiled, or in need of straightening. Bed linens must be changed frequently for these reasons:

- Sheets that are damp, wrinkled, or bunched up under a client are uncomfortable. They may prevent the client from resting or sleeping well.

- Microorganisms thrive in moist, warm environments. Bedding that is damp or unclean encourages infection and disease.

- Clients who spend long hours in bed are at risk for pressure sores. Sheets that do not lie flat under the client's body increase the risk of pressure sores because they cut off circulation.

If a client cannot get out of bed, you must change the linens with the client in bed. An occupied bed is made with the client in bed. When making the bed, use a wide stance. Bend your knees. Avoid bending from the waist, especially when tucking sheets or blankets under the mattress. Mattresses can be heavy, so remember to bend your knees to avoid injury. It is easier to make an empty bed than one with a client in it. An unoccupied bed is a bed made while no client is in the bed. If the client can be moved, your job will be easier.

Making an occupied bed

Equipment: clean linen—mattress pad, fitted or flat bottom sheet, waterproof bed protector if needed, cotton draw sheet, flat top sheet, blanket(s), bath blanket, pillowcase(s), gloves

1. Wash your hands.

2. Explain the procedure to the client, speaking clearly, slowly, and directly. Maintain face-to-face contact whenever possible.

3. Provide privacy if the client desires it.

4. Place clean linen on clean surface within reach (e.g., bedside stand or chair).

5. If the bed is adjustable, adjust bed to a safe working level, usually waist high. Lower the head of the bed. If the bed is movable, lock bed wheels.

6. Put on gloves.

7. Loosen top linen from the end of the bed on the working side. Unfold the bath blanket over the top sheet to cover the client, and remove the top sheet.

8. You will make the bed one side at a time. If the bed has side rails, raise side rail on far side of bed. This protects the client from falling out of the bed while you are making it. After

raising the side rail, go to the other side. Assist the client to turn onto her side, moving away from you toward the raised side rail.

9. Loosen the bottom soiled linen, mattress pad, and protector, if present, on the working side.

10. Roll bottom soiled linen toward client, tucking it snugly against the client's back.

11. Place and tuck in clean bottom linen, finishing with bottom sheet free of wrinkles. If you are using a flat bottom sheet, leave enough overlap on each end to tuck under the mattress. If the sheet is only long enough to tuck in at one end, tuck it in securely at the top of the bed. Make hospital corners to keep bottom sheet wrinkle-free (Fig. 6-2).

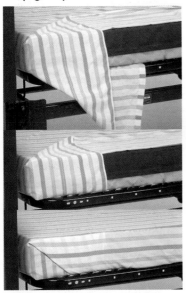

Fig. 6-2. Hospital corners help keep the flat sheet smooth under the client. They help prevent the feet from being restricted by or tangled in linen when getting in and out of bed.

12. Smooth the bottom sheet out toward the client. Be sure there are no wrinkles in the mattress pad. Roll the extra material toward the client and tuck it under the client's body.

13. If using a waterproof pad, unfold it and center it on the bed. Tuck the side near you under the mattress. Smooth it out toward the client, and tuck as you did with the sheet.

14. If using a draw sheet, place it on the bed. Tuck in on your side, smooth, and tuck as you did with the other bedding.

15. Raise side rail nearest you. Go to the other side of the bed and lower the side rail on that side. Assist client to turn onto clean bottom sheet. Protect the client from any soiled matter on the old linens.

16. Loosen the soiled linen. Check for any personal items. Roll linen from head to the foot of bed. Avoid contact with your skin or clothes. Place it in a hamper or basket. Never put it on the floor or furniture. Never shake it. Soiled bed linens are full of microorganisms that should not be spread to other parts of the room.

17. Pull and tuck in clean bottom linen just like the other side, finishing with bottom sheet free of wrinkles.

18. Ask client to turn onto her back. Keep client covered and comfortable, with a pillow under the head. Raise the side rail.

19. Unfold the top sheet and place it over the client. Ask the client to hold the top sheet. Slip the blanket or old sheet out from

underneath. Put it in the laundry hamper.

20. Place a blanket over the top sheet, matching the top edges. Tuck the bottom edges of top sheet and blanket under the bottom of the mattress. Make hospital corners on each side. Loosen the top linens over the client's feet. This prevents pressure on the feet. At the top of the bed, fold the top sheet over the blanket about six inches.

21. Remove the pillow. Do not hold it near your face. Remove the soiled pillowcase by turning it inside out. Place it in the laundry hamper.

22. Remove and discard gloves. Wash your hands.

23. With one hand, grasp the clean pillowcase at the closed end. Turn it inside out over your arm. Next, using the same hand that has the pillowcase over it, grasp one narrow edge of the pillow. Pull the pillowcase over it with your free hand (Fig. 6-3). Do the same for any

other pillows. Place them under your client's head or as client desires.

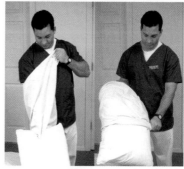

Fig. 6-3. *After the pillowcase is turned inside out over your arm, grasp one end of the pillow. Pull the pillowcase over the pillow.*

24. If you raised an adjustable bed, be sure to return it to its lowest position. Leave side rails in the ordered position. Put any signaling device within the client's reach. Carry laundry hamper to laundry area.

25. Wash your hands.

26. Document the procedure and any observations.

Making an unoccupied bed

Equipment: clean linen—mattress pad, fitted or flat bottom sheet, waterproof bed protector if needed, cotton draw sheet, flat top sheet, blanket(s), pillowcase(s), gloves

1. Wash your hands.

2. Place clean linen on clean surface within reach (e.g., bedside stand or chair).

3. If the bed is adjustable, adjust bed to a safe working level, usually waist high. Put bed in flattest position. If the bed is movable, lock bed wheels.

4. Put on gloves.

5. Loosen soiled linen. Roll soiled linen (soiled side inside) from head to foot of bed. Avoid contact with your skin or clothes. Place it in a hamper or basket

6. Remove and discard gloves. Wash your hands.

7. Remake the bed, spreading mattress pad and bottom sheet, tucking under mattress. Make hospital corners to keep bottom sheet wrinkle-free. Put on mattress protector and draw

sheet. Smooth and tuck under sides of bed.

8. Place top sheet and blanket over bed. Center these, tuck under end of bed, and make hospital corners. Fold down the top sheet over the blanket about six inches. Fold both top sheet and blanket down so client can easily get into bed. If client will not be returning to bed immediately, leave bedding up.

9. Remove pillows and pillowcases. Put on clean pillowcases (as described in procedure above). Replace pillows.

10. If you raised an adjustable bed, be sure to return it to its lowest position.

11. Carry laundry hamper to laundry area.

12. Wash your hands.

13. Document the procedure and any observations.

Proper Nutrition

Nutrition

Good nutrition is very important. Nutrition is how the body uses food to maintain health. Bodies need a well-balanced diet containing essential nutrients and plenty of fluids. This helps us grow new cells, maintain normal body function, and have energy. Good nutrition in early life helps ensure good health later in life. For those who are ill or elderly, a well-balanced diet helps maintain muscle and skin tissues and prevent pressure sores. A good diet promotes healing. It also helps us cope with stress.

A nutrient is something found in food that provides energy, promotes growth and health, and helps regulate metabolism. Metabolism is the process by which nutrients are broken down to be used by the body for energy and other needs. The body needs the following six nutrients for growth and development:

1. **Protein**: Proteins are part of every body cell. They are essential for tissue growth and repair. Proteins also supply energy for the body. Excess proteins are excreted by the kidneys or stored as body fat. Sources of protein include fish, seafood, poultry, meat, eggs, milk, cheese, nuts, nut butters, peas, dried beans or legumes, and soy products (tofu, tempeh, veggie burgers). Whole grain cereals, pastas, rice, and breads contain some proteins, too.

2. **Carbohydrates**: Carbohydrates supply the fuel for the body's energy needs. They supply extra protein and help the body use fat efficiently. Carbohydrates also provide fiber, which is necessary for bowel elimination. Carbohydrates can be divided into two basic types: complex and simple carbohydrates. Complex carbohydrates are found in bread, cereal, potatoes, rice, pasta, vegetables, and fruits. Simple carbohy-

drates are found in sugars, sweets, syrups, and jellies. Simple carbohydrates do not have the same nutritional value as complex carbohydrates do.

3. **Fats**: Fat helps the body store energy. Body fat also provides the body
with insulation. It protects body organs. In addition, fats add flavor to
food and are important for the absorption of certain vitamins. Excess
fat in the diet is stored as fat in the body. Examples of fats are butter,
margarine, salad dressings, oils, and animal fats found in meats, fowl,
and fish. Monounsaturated vegetable fats (including olive oil and
canola oil) and polyunsaturated vegetable fats (including corn and saf-
flower oils) are healthier kinds of fats. Saturated fats, including animal
fats like butter, lard, bacon and other fatty meats, are not as healthy.
They should be limited in most diets.

4. **Vitamins**: Vitamins are substances the body needs to function. The
body cannot produce most vitamins. They can only be obtained from
food. Vitamins A, D, E, and K are fat-soluble vitamins. This means
they are carried and stored in body fat. Vitamins B and C are water-sol-
uble vitamins that are broken down by water in our bodies. They cannot be stored in the body. They are eliminated in urine and feces.

5. **Minerals**: Minerals form and maintain body functions. They provide
energy and control processes. Zinc, iron, calcium, and magnesium are
examples of minerals. Minerals are found in many foods.

6. **Water**: Because one-half to two-thirds of our body weight is water, we
need about 64 ounces, or eight 8-ounce glasses, of water or other fluids a day. Water is the most essential nutrient for life. Without it, a person can only live a few days. Water assists in the digestion and absorption of food. It helps with waste elimination. Through perspiration,
water also helps maintain normal body temperature. Maintaining fluid
balance in our bodies is necessary for good health.

The fluids we drink—water, juice, soda, coffee, tea, and milk—provide
most of the water our bodies use. Some foods are also sources of water,
including soup, celery, lettuce, apples, and peaches.

Most foods contain several nutrients, but no one food contains all the
nutrients needed for a healthy body. This is why it is important to eat a
daily diet that is well-balanced. There is not one single dietary plan that is
right for everyone. People have different nutritional needs, depending
upon their age, gender, and activity level.

In 1980, the U.S. Department of Agriculture (USDA) developed the Food
Guide Pyramid to help promote healthy eating practices. In 2005, in
response to new scientific information about nutrition and health and

new technology for support tools, MyPyramid was developed (Fig. 6-4). MyPyramid replaces the Food Guide Pyramid. MyPyramid is a personalized version of the Food Guide Pyramid that offers individual plans based on age, gender, and activity level.

The Pyramid is made up of six bands of different widths and colors. Each color represents a food group—orange for grains, green for vegetables, maroon for fruits, yellow for oils, blue for milk, and purple for meat and beans. The different widths indicate that not all groups should make up an equal part of a healthy diet. The orange band, grains, is the widest. This means that grains should make up the highest proportion of the diet. The smaller bands, such as the purple band representing meat and beans, should make up a smaller part of foods eaten. The smallest band, the yellow one, represents oils. Oils contain essential fatty acids. However, this band is not emphasized because the body needs fats and oils in smaller quantities.

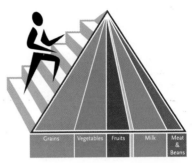

Fig. 6-4. *MyPyramid was developed to help promote healthy eating practices. It offers individual plans based on age, gender and activity level.*

The bands of the Pyramid are wide at the bottom and narrow into a point at the top. This is a reminder that there are a great variety of foods that make up each group. Many choices are available to help meet the daily requirements. Foods that are nutrient-dense and low in fat and calories should form the "base" of a healthy diet. They are represented by the wide base of the Pyramid. Foods that are high in fat and sugar and have less nutritional value are at the narrow top. They should be eaten less often.

The new Pyramid also emphasizes the importance of physical activity, as represented by the figure climbing the stairs. Physical activity goes hand-in-hand with diet to make up an overall healthy lifestyle. The USDA recommends at least 30 minutes per day of vigorous activity for everyone. Sixty minutes or more is even better.

Grains: The grains group includes all foods made from wheat, rice, oats, corn, barley, and other grains. Examples are bread, pasta, oatmeal, breakfast cereals, tortillas, and grits. One slice of bread, one cup of ready-to-eat cereal, or ½ cup of cooked rice, pasta, or cooked cereal can be counted as a one-ounce equivalent from the grains group. At least half of all grains consumed should be whole grains. Words on food labels that ensure that grains are whole grains are: brown rice, wild rice, bulgur, oatmeal, whole-grain corn, whole oats, whole wheat, and whole rye. Words that do not usually indicate whole grains include: multi-grain, stone-ground, 100% wheat, cracked wheat, seven-grain, or bran.

Vegetables: The vegetable group includes all fresh, frozen, canned and dried vegetables and vegetable juices. One cup of raw or cooked vegetables or vegetable juice or two cups of raw leafy greens can be counted as one cup from the vegetable group. There are five subgroups within the vegetable group. They are organized by nutritional content. These are dark green vegetables, orange vegetables, dry beans and peas, starchy vegetables, and other vegetables. A variety of vegetables from these subgroups should be eaten every day. Dark green vegetables, orange vegetables, and dried beans and peas have the best nutritional content. Vegetables are low in fat and calories and have no cholesterol (although sauces and seasonings may add fat, calories, and cholesterol). They are good sources of dietary fiber, potassium, vitamin A, vitamin E, and vitamin C.

Fruits: The fruit group includes all fresh, frozen, canned and dried fruits and fruit juices. One cup of fruit or 100% fruit juice or ½ cup of dried fruit can be counted as one cup from the fruit group. Most choices should be whole or cut up fruit, rather than juice, for the additional dietary fiber provided. Fruits, like vegetables, are naturally low in fat, sodium and calories and have no cholesterol. They are important sources of dietary fiber and many nutrients, including folic acid and vitamin C.

Milk: The milk group includes all fluid milk products and foods made from milk that retain their calcium content, such as yogurt and cheese. Foods made from milk that have little to no calcium, such as cream cheese, cream, and butter, are not part of the group. Most milk group choices should be fat-free or low-fat. One cup of milk or yogurt, one and a half ounces of natural cheese, or two ounces of processed cheese can be counted as one cup from the milk group. Foods in the milk group provide nutrients that are vital for the health and maintenance of your body. These nutrients include calcium, potassium, vitamin D, and protein. Calcium is used for building bones and teeth and in maintaining bone mass. Milk products are the primary source of calcium in American diets.

Meat and Beans: One ounce of lean meat, poultry, or fish, one egg, one tablespoon of peanut butter, ¼ cup cooked dry beans, or ½ ounce of nuts or seeds can be counted as one-ounce equivalent from the meat and beans group. Dry beans and peas can be included as part of this group or part of the vegetable group. If meat is eaten regularly, they should be included with vegetables. If not, they should be included in this group.

Most meat and poultry choices should be lean or low-fat. Diets that are high in saturated fats raise "bad" cholesterol levels in the blood. Some food choices in this group are high in saturated fat. These include fatty cuts of beef, pork, and lamb; regular (75% to 85% lean) ground beef; regular sausages, hot dogs, and bacon; some luncheon meats, such as regular bologna and salami; and some poultry, such as duck. These foods should be limited to help keep blood cholesterol levels healthy. Fish, nuts, and seeds contain healthy oils. These foods are a good choice instead of meat or poultry. Some nuts and seeds (flax, walnuts) are excellent sources of essential fatty acids. These acids may reduce the risk of cardiovascular disease. Some (sunflower seeds, almonds, hazelnuts) are good sources of vitamin E.

Vegetarians get enough protein from this group as long as the variety and amounts of foods selected are adequate. Protein sources for vegetarians from this group include eggs (for ovo-vegetarians), beans, nuts, nut butters, peas, and soy products (tofu, tempeh, veggie burgers).

Oils: Oils include fats that are liquid at room temperature, such as canola, corn, olive, soybean, and sunflower oil. Some foods are naturally high in oils, like nuts, olives, some fish, and avocados. Foods that are mainly oil include mayonnaise, certain salad dressings, and soft margarine. Most of the fats you eat should be polyunsaturated (PUFA) or monounsaturated (MUFA) fats. Oils are the major source of MUFAs and PUFAs in the diet. PUFAs contain some fatty acids that are necessary for health. These are called "essential fatty acids." Most Americans consume enough oil in the foods they eat, such as nuts, fish, cooking oil, and salad dressings.

Activity: Physical activity and nutrition work together for better health. Being active increases the amount of calories burned. As people age, their metabolism slows. Maintaining energy balance requires moving more and eating less. For health benefits, physical activity should be moderate or vigorous and add up to at least 30 minutes a day. For more information on MyPyramid, visit mypyramid.gov.

Older adults have different nutritional needs. Tufts University developed a version of MyPyramid that is specifically designed for older adults. Due to slower metabolism and less activity, the elderly need to eat less to maintain body weight. Although calories can be reduced, daily needs for most nutrients do not decrease. The "Modified MyPyramid for Older Adults" has a narrower base to reflect a decrease in energy needs. It emphasizes nutrient-dense foods, fiber, and water. Dietary supplements may be appropriate for many older people. For more information on the "Modified MyPyramid for Older Adults," visit nutrition.tufts.edu.

Most clients should be encouraged to drink at least 64 ounces of water or other fluids a day. Remember that water is essential for life. The sense of thirst often diminishes as people age. Remind your elderly clients to drink fluids often. Some clients will drink more fluids if they are offered to them in smaller amounts. However, some clients may have an order to restrict fluids (RF) or to force fluids (FF) because of medical conditions. Follow your client's care plan.

Dehydration occurs when a person does not have enough fluid in the body. Dehydration is a serious condition. People can become dehydrated if they do not drink enough or if they have diarrhea or are vomiting. Preventing dehydration is very important.

Observing and Reporting: Dehydration

Report any of these to your supervisor:

O/R Client drinks less than eight 8-ounce glasses of liquid per day.

O/R Client drinks little or no fluids at meals.

O/R Client needs help drinking from a cup or glass.

O/R Client has trouble swallowing liquids.

O/R Client has frequent vomiting, diarrhea, or fever.

O/R Client is easily tired or confused.

Report any of these symptoms:

O/R Dry mouth

O/R Cracked lips

O/R Sunken eyes

O/R Dark urine

O/R Strong-smelling urine

O/R Weight loss

O/R Complaints of abdominal pain

Guidelines: Preventing Dehydration

G Report observations and warning signs to your supervisor immediately.

G Encourage your clients to drink every time you see them.

G Offer fresh water or other fluids often. Offer drinks that client enjoys. Some may not like water and prefer other types of beverages, such as juice, soda, tea, or milk. Some may not want ice in their drinks. Honor personal preferences.

G   Record fluid intake and output if assigned.

G   Ice chips, frozen flavored ice sticks, and gelatin are also forms of liquids. Offer them often. Do not offer ice chips or sticks if a client has a swallowing problem.

G   If appropriate, offer sips of liquid between bites of food at meals and during snack time.

G   Make sure a pitcher and cup are close enough and light enough for a client to lift.

G   Offer assistance if a client cannot drink without help. Use adaptive cups as needed.

Fluid overload occurs when the body cannot handle the amount of fluid consumed. This condition often affects people with heart or kidney disease.

Observing and Reporting: Fluid Overload

O/R   Swelling/edema of extremities (ankles, feet, fingers, hands)

O/R   Weight gain (daily weight gain of one to two pounds)

O/R   Less urine output

O/R   Shortness of breath

O/R   Increased heart rate

O/R   Skin that appears tight, smooth, and shiny

Aging and illness can lead to emotional and physical problems that affect the intake of food. For example, people who are lonely or who suffer from illnesses that affect their ability to chew and swallow may have little interest in food.

Unintended weight loss is a serious problem for the elderly. Weight loss can mean that the client has a serious medical condition. It can lead to skin breakdown, which leads to pressure sores. It is very important to report any weight loss you notice, no matter how small.

Observing and Reporting: Unintended Weight Loss

Report any of these to your supervisor:

O/R   Client needs help eating or drinking

O/R   Client eats less than 70% of meals/snacks served

O/R   Client has mouth pain

O/R   Client has dentures that do not fit properly

O/R   Client has any difficulty chewing or swallowing

O/R   Client coughs or chokes while eating

O/R   Client is sad, has crying spells, or withdraws from others

O/R   Client is confused, wanders, or paces

Guidelines: Preventing Unintended Weight Loss

G   Report observations and warning signs to your supervisor.

G   Encourage clients to eat. Talk about food served in a positive tone of voice. Use positive words.

G   Honor clients' food likes and dislikes.

G   Offer different kinds of foods and beverages.

G   Help clients who have trouble feeding themselves.

G   Food should look, taste, and smell good. The person may have a poor sense of taste and smell.

G   Season foods to clients' preferences.

G   Allow enough time for clients to finish eating.

G   Notify your supervisor if clients have trouble using utensils.

G   Record the meal/snack intake if assigned.

G   Provide oral care before and after meals, if the client requests it.

G   Position clients sitting upright for feeding.

G   If a client has had a loss of appetite and/or seems sad, ask about it.

Clients with swallowing problems may be restricted to consuming only thickened liquids. Thickening improves the ability to control fluid in the mouth and throat. A doctor orders the necessary thickness after the client has been evaluated by a speech therapist. If thickening is ordered, it must be used with all liquids. You need to know what thickened liquids mean. Do not offer these clients regular liquids. Do not offer water or other beverages to a client who must have thickened liquids.

Follow the directions for each client as listed in the care plan. Three basic thickened consistencies are:

1. **Nectar Thick**: This consistency is thicker than water. It is the thickness of a thick juice, such as pear nectar or tomato juice. A client can drink this from a cup.

2. **Honey Thick**: This consistency has the thickness of honey. It will pour very slowly. A client will usually use a spoon to consume it.

3. **Pudding Thick**: With this consistency, the liquids have become semi-solid, much like pudding. A spoon should stand up straight in the glass when put into the middle of the drink. A client must consume these liquids with a spoon.

Swallowing problems put clients at high risk for choking on food or drink. Inhaling food, fluid, or foreign material into the lungs is called aspiration. Aspiration can cause pneumonia or death. Notify your supervisor immediately if any problems occur while feeding.

Guidelines: Preventing Aspiration

G   Position clients properly when eating. They must sit in a straight, upright position. Do not try to feed clients in a reclining position.

G   Offer small pieces of food or small spoons of pureed food.

G   Feed clients slowly.

G   Place food in the non-paralyzed, or unaffected, side of the mouth.

G   Make sure mouth is empty before each bite of food or sip of drink.

G   Clients should stay in the upright position for about 30 minutes after eating and drinking.

When the digestive system does not function properly, hyperalimentation or total parenteral nutrition (TPN) may be needed. With TPN, a client receives nutrients directly into the bloodstream. It bypasses the digestive system.

When a person is unable to swallow, he or she may be fed through a tube. A nasogastric tube is inserted into the nose and goes to the stomach. A tube can also be placed through the skin directly into the stomach. This is called a percutaneous endoscopic gastrostomy (PEG) tube. The opening in the stomach and abdomen is called a gastrostomy (Fig. 6-5). Tube feedings are used when clients cannot swallow but can digest food.

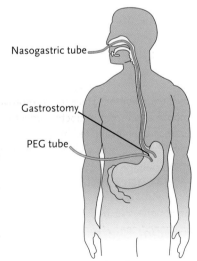

Fig. 6-5. Nasogastric tubes are inserted through the nose. PEG tubes are inserted through the skin directly into the stomach.

Home health aides are not responsible for tube or TPN feedings. HHAs do not insert or remove tubes, do the feeding, or clean the tubes. You may be assigned to take the person's temperature or assemble equipment and supplies. You may also discard or clean used equipment and supplies. In addition, you should observe, report, and document any changes in the client or problems with the feeding.

When planning meals and cooking for your clients, know their food preferences. Some of these may be listed in the care plan. You will also need to find out more before planning meals. Ask the client or a family member to tell you about food preferences, or suggest some sample menus and ask for reactions. Pay attention to what is eaten when you serve meals. If a client never finishes her chicken, it may mean that she prefers other kinds of meats. Cost may also be a factor in choosing foods. Protein-rich foods are generally the most expensive, but also the most important for the healing process.

The Food and Drug Administration (FDA) requires that all packaged foods contain a standardized nutrition label, called "Nutrition Facts" (Fig. 6-6) The Nutrition Facts label gives you the following information:

- Serving size and number of servings per container

- Calories per serving and calories from fat per serving

- How much a serving contains and the percentage of the recommended daily total a serving contains

- Percentage of recommended daily totals for certain vitamins and minerals

Regular Frozen Lasagna

Nutrition Facts
Serving size 1 Package (10.75 oz.)

Amount Per Serving

Calories 360   **Calories from Fat** 120

	% Daily Value
Total Fat 13g	20%
Saturated Fat 7g	35%
Cholesterol 35mg	11%
Sodium 960mg *high*	40%
Total Carbohydrate 40g	14%
Dietary Fiber 6g	23%
Sugars 10g	
Protein 21g	

Calcium	35%
Vitamin A	10%
Vitamin C	10%
Iron	6%

Fig. 6-6. The FDA-required Nutrition Facts label contains standard nutritional information that makes it easier to compare different products.

Special Diets

A doctor sometimes places clients who are ill on special diets. These diets are known as "therapeutic," "modified," or "special" diets. Certain nutrients or fluids may be restricted. Medications may interact with certain foods, which then need to be eliminated. Doctors may order special diets for clients who do not eat enough. Diets are also prescribed for weight control and food allergies.

You will play an important role in helping clients follow their modified diets. The care plan should specify any special diet the client is on. Never modify a client's diet. Therapeutic diets can only be prescribed by doctors and planned by dietitians. Follow the client's diet plan.

Low-Sodium Diet: People are most familiar with sodium as one of the two ingredients of salt. Salt is the first food to be restricted in a low-sodium diet because it is high in sodium. Foods high in sodium include cured meats: ham, bacon, lunch meat, sausage, salt pork, and hot dogs; salty or smoked fish: herring, salted cod, sardines, anchovies, caviar, smoked salmon or lox; processed cheese; canned and dried soups; vegetables preserved in brine: pickles, sauerkraut, olives, relishes; salted foods: nuts, dips, and spreads; sauces with high concentrations of salt: Worcestershire, barbecue, chili, and soy sauces; ketchup, mustard, and mayonnaise; canned foods; some cereals; gelatin desserts; and over-the-counter medications and drugs.

For clients on a low-sodium diet, read product labels to determine if they contain salt or sodium in any form. You can make low-sodium meals more flavorful by adding lemon, herbs, dry mustard, pepper, paprika, orange rind, onion, and garlic to recipes. The flavor of meats can also be enhanced by the addition of fruits and jellies.

Common abbreviations for this diet are "Low Na," which means low sodium, or "NAS," which stands for "No Added Salt."

Fluid-Restricted Diet: The fluid taken into the body through food and fluids must equal the amount of fluid that leaves the body through perspiration, stool, urine, and expiration. This is fluid balance. When fluid intake is greater than fluid output, body tissues become swollen with fluid. In addition, people with severe heart disease and kidney disease may have trouble processing fluid. To prevent further damage, doctors may restrict fluid intake. For clients on fluid restriction, you will need to measure and document exact amounts of fluid intake. Report excesses to your supervisor. Do not offer additional fluids or foods that count as fluids, such as ice cream, puddings, gelatin, etc. If the client complains of thirst or requests fluids, tell your supervisor. A common abbreviation for this diet is "RF," which stands for "Restrict Fluids."

High-Potassium Diet (K+): Some clients are on diuretics, which are medications that reduce fluid volume, or on blood pressure medications. These clients may be excreting so much fluid that their bodies could be depleted of potassium. Other clients may be placed on a high-potassium diet for different reasons.

Foods high in potassium include bananas, grapefruit, oranges, orange juice, prune juice, prunes, dried apricots, figs, raisins, dates, cantaloupes, tomatoes, potatoes with skins, sweet potatoes and yams, winter squash, legumes, avocados, and unsalted nuts. "K+" is the common abbreviation for this diet.

Low-Protein Diet: People who have kidney disease may be on low-protein diets. Protein is restricted because it breaks down into compounds that may further damage the kidneys. The extent of the restriction depends on the stage of the disease and if the client is on dialysis. Exchange lists show foods that can be exchanged for one another on a meal plan. They are used extensively in special diets for people with diabetes. Exchange lists have also been developed for clients on diets modified for protein, potassium, and sodium. Follow the instructions for these diets carefully and ask for help whenever you need it.

Low-Fat/Low-Cholesterol Diet: People who have high levels of cholesterol in their blood are at risk for heart attacks and heart disease. People with gallbladder disease, diseases that interfere with fat digestion, and liver disease are also placed on low-fat/low-cholesterol diets. Low-fat/low-cholesterol diets permit skim milk, low-fat cottage cheese, fish, white meat of turkey and chicken, veal, and vegetable fats (especially monounsaturated fats such as olive, canola, and peanut oils). Clients may be advised to limit their diets in these ways:

- Eat lean cuts of meat, including lamb, beef, and pork, and eat these only three times a week.
- Limit egg yolks to three or four per week (including eggs used in baking).
- Avoid organ meats, shellfish, fatty meats, cream, butter, lard, meat drippings, coconut and palm oils, and desserts and soups made with whole milk.
- Avoid fried foods and sweets.

People who have gallbladder disease or other digestive problems may be placed on a diet that restricts all fats. A common abbreviation for this diet is "Low-Fat/Low-Chol."

Modified Calorie Diet: Some clients may need to reduce calories to lose weight or prevent additional weight gain. Other clients need to increase calories because of malnutrition, surgery, illness, or fever. Clients with certain conditions need more protein to promote growth and repair of tissue and regulation of body functions. Common abbreviations for this diet are "Low-Cal" or "High-Cal."

Bland Diet: Gastric and duodenal ulcers can be irritated by foods that produce or increase levels of acid in the stomach. People who have ulcers usually know the foods that cause them discomfort. Doctors will advise them to avoid these foods as well as the following: alcohol; beverages containing caffeine, such as coffee, tea, and soft drinks; citrus juices; spicy foods; and spicy seasonings, such as black pepper, cayenne, and chili pepper. Three meals or more a day are usually advised. If alcohol is allowed, it should be consumed with meals.

Dietary Management of Diabetes: People with diabetes must be very careful about what they eat. Calories and carbohydrates are carefully controlled in the diets of diabetic clients. Protein and fats are also regulated. The foods and the amounts are determined by nutritional and energy needs. See Part V for more information on diabetes.

A dietitian and the client will make up a meal plan together. It will include all the right types and amounts of food for each day. The client uses exchange lists, or lists of similar foods that can be substituted for one another, to make up a menu. Using meal plans and exchange lists, a person with diabetes can control his diet while still making food choices. To keep their blood glucose levels near normal, diabetic clients must eat the right amount of the right type of food at the right time. They must eat all that is served. Encourage them to do so. Do not offer other foods without the doctor's approval. If a client will not eat what is directed, or if you think that he or she is not following the diet, inform your supervisor.

Diabetics should avoid foods that are high in sugar, such as candy, because sugary foods can cause problems with insulin balance. Foods and drinks high in sugar include candy, ice cream, cakes, cookies, jellies, jams, fruits canned in heavy syrup, soft drinks, and alcoholic beverages. Many foods are high in sugar that do not appear to be so, such as canned fruits and vegetables, many breakfast cereals, and ketchup.

The common abbreviations for this diet are "NCS," which stands for "No Concentrated Sweets" or the allowed amount of calories followed by the abbreviation "ADA," which stands for American Diabetic Association.

Low-Residue (Low-Fiber) Diet: This diet decreases the amount of fiber, whole grains, raw fruits and vegetables, seeds, and other foods, such as dairy and coffee. The low-residue diet is used for people with bowel disturbances.

High-Residue (High-Fiber) Diet: High-residue diets increase the intake of fiber and whole grains, such as whole grain cereals, bread, and raw fruits and vegetables. This diet helps with problems such as constipation and bowel disorders.

Diets may also be modified in consistency:

Liquid Diet: A liquid diet is usually ordered for a short time. It may be ordered due to a medical condition or before or after a test or surgery. A liquid diet is made up of foods that are in a liquid state at body temperature. Liquid diets are usually ordered as "clear" or "full." A clear liquid diet includes clear juices, broth, gelatin, and popsicles. A full liquid diet includes clear liquids with the addition of cream soups, milk, and ice cream.

Soft Diet and Mechanical Soft Diet: The soft diet is soft in texture and consists of soft or chopped foods that are easier to chew and swallow. Foods that are hard to chew and swallow, such as raw fruits and vegetables and some meats, will be restricted. High-fiber foods, fried foods, and spicy foods may also be limited to help with digestion. Doctors order this diet for residents who have trouble chewing and swallowing due to dental problems or other medical conditions. It is also ordered for people who are making the transition from a liquid diet to a regular diet.

The mechanical soft diet consists of chopped or blended foods that are easier to chew and swallow. Foods are prepared with blenders, food processors, or cutting utensils. Unlike the soft diet, the mechanical soft diet does not limit spices, fat, and fiber. Only the texture of foods is changed. For example, meats and poultry can be ground and moistened with sauces or water to ease swallowing. This diet is used for people recovering from surgery or who have difficulty chewing and swallowing.

Pureed Diet: To puree a food means to chop, blend, or grind it into a thick paste of baby food consistency. The food should be thick enough to hold its form in the mouth. This diet does not require a person to chew his or her food. A pureed diet is often used for people who have trouble chewing and/or swallowing more textured foods.

Planning and Shopping

It is very important to plan meals for a week or at least several days before shopping. When your meal plan is completed, make your shopping list. On a large sheet of paper, write down categories, including produce, meats, canned goods, frozen foods, dairy, and other. Leave space under each category to list the foods you need to buy. Listing items by category will save you time in the grocery store. Go through your plan meal by meal. Write down all of the ingredients you will need for each meal. Remember to include beverages. Check the refrigerator, cabinets, and pantry for ingredients. Many ingredients you need may already be in the home. Keep a shopping list going all the time so family members, clients, and you can write down things you run out of during the week.

Guidelines: Shopping for Clients

G Use coupons. If your client receives a newspaper, scan it for coupons from stores or manufacturers. Clip and use only those coupons for items you have already planned to buy.

G Check store circulars for advertised specials.

G Buy fresh foods that are in season, when they are at peak flavor and inexpensive.

G Buy in quantity. Large amounts or larger sizes are usually more economical, but do not buy more than you can store.

G Shop from your list. Do not be tempted by items that are not on your list.

G Avoid processed, already-mixed, or ready-made foods. They are usually more expensive and less nutritious. When time allows, buy staples, or basic items.

G Loaves of bread are generally a better buy than rolls or crackers. Day-old bread is usually sold at reduced prices.

G Milk can be bought in many forms. Choose the type that the client prefers. Skim, one percent, or two percent milk contains lower fat and is usually cheaper than whole milk.

G Buy a cheaper brand when appearance is not important.

G Read labels to be sure you are getting the kind of product and the quantity you want.

G Estimate the cost per serving before buying. Divide the total cost by the number of servings to determine the cost per serving.

G Consider the amount of waste in bones and fat when buying cheaper cuts of meat.

G Avoid convenience stores. Shopping at large supermarkets or discount stores usually guarantees you will get the best prices.

G Plan ahead. Knowing what you need and buying before you run out will save you money.

When deciding what to buy, keep these four factors in mind:

1. Nutritional value

2. Quality

3. Price

4. Preference

Preparing and Storing

Food-borne illnesses affect up to 100 million people each year. Elderly people are at increased risk partly because they may not see, smell, or taste that food is spoiled. They also may not have the energy to prepare and store food safely. For people who have weakened immune systems because of AIDS or cancer, a food-borne illness can be deadly.

Guidelines: Safe Food Preparation

G   Wash hands frequently. Wash your hands thoroughly before beginning any food preparation. Wash your hands after handling raw meat, poultry, or fish.

G   Keep your hair tied back or covered. Wear clean clothes or a clean apron.

G   Wear gloves when you have a cut or wound on your hands.

G   Avoid coughing or sneezing around food. If you cough or sneeze, wash your hands immediately.

G   Keep everything clean. Clean and disinfect countertops and other surfaces before, during (as necessary), and after food preparation.

G   Handle raw meat, poultry, and fish carefully. Use an antibacterial kitchen cleaner or a dilute bleach solution to clean any countertops on which meat juices have spilled. Wrap paper or packaging containing meat juices in plastic and discard immediately.

G   Once you have used a knife or cutting board to cut fresh meat, do not use it for anything else until it has been washed in hot soapy water, rinsed in clear water, and allowed to air dry.

G   Use one cutting board for raw meat, poultry, and seafood, and a separate cutting board for fresh produce and bread.

G   Use hot, soapy water to wash utensils.

G   Change dishcloths, sponges, and towels frequently. Sponges may be washed in the dishwasher to disinfect them.

G   Defrost frozen foods in the refrigerator, not on the countertop. Do not remove meats or dairy products from the refrigerator until just before use.

G   Wash fruits and vegetables thoroughly in running water to remove pesticides and bacteria.

G   Cook meats, poultry, and fish thoroughly to kill any harmful microorganisms they may contain. Heat leftovers thoroughly. Never leave food out for over two hours. Keep cold foods cold and hot foods hot.

G   Do not use cracked eggs. Do not consume or serve raw eggs.

G   Never taste and stir with the same utensil.

The following basic methods of food preparation will allow you to prepare a variety of healthy meals:

Boiling: Food is cooked in boiling water until tender or done. This is the
best method for cooking pasta, noodles, rice, and hard- or soft-boiled
eggs.

Steaming: Steaming is a healthy
way to prepare vegetables. A small
amount of water is boiled in the
bottom of a saucepan and food is
set over it on a rack. The pan is
tightly covered to keep the steam in
(Fig. 6-7).

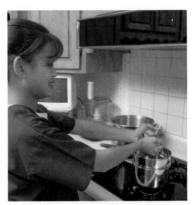

Poaching: Fish or eggs may be
cooked by poaching in barely boiling water or other liquid. Eggs are
cracked and shells discarded before
poaching. Fish may be poached in
milk or broth, on top of the stove or
in the oven in a baking dish.

Fig. 6-7. *Steaming allows vegetables
to retain their vitamins and flavor.*

Roasting: Used for meats and poultry or some vegetables, roasting is a
simple way to cook. Dry heat roasting means food is roasted in an open
pan in the oven. Meats and poultry are basted, or coated with juices or
other liquid, during roasting.

Braising: Braising is a slow-cooking method that uses moist heat. Liquid
such as broth, wine, or tomato sauce is poured over and around meat or
vegetables, and the pot is covered. The meat or vegetables are then slowly cooked at a temperature just below boiling. Braising is a good way to
tenderize tough meats and vegetables, since the long cooking breaks
down their fibers. Braising may be done in the oven or on the stove top.

Baking: Baking is used for many foods, including breads, poultry, fish,
and vegetables. Baking is done at a moderate heat, 350°F to 400°F.
Vegetables such as potatoes and winter squash bake very well.

Broiling: Used primarily for meats, broiling involves cooking food close to the source of heat at a high temperature for a short time. Meat must be tender to be broiled successfully. Inexpensive and lean cuts are often better cooked using moist heat. The "broil" setting on the oven can also be used to melt cheese or brown the top of a casserole. Leave the oven door ajar when broiling and never leave the kitchen; things can burn very fast.

slightly open

Sautéing or stir-frying: These are quick cooking methods for vegetables and meats. Use a small amount of oil in a frying pan or wok over high heat.

Microwaving: Microwave ovens are safe to use for defrosting, reheating, and cooking. However, "cold spots" can occur in microwaved foods. To minimize cold spots, stir and rotate the food once or twice during cooking. Place food in microwave-safe bowls before cooking. To ensure that meat is properly cooked, use a meat thermometer. This verifies that the food has reached a safe temperature. Never place metal thermometers or any metal object in microwaves.

Frying: Frying uses a lot of fat and is the least healthy way to cook. Avoid frying foods for clients.

Fresh, uncooked foods: Many fruits and vegetables have the most nutrients when eaten fresh, as in salads (Fig. 6-8). However, fresh fruits and vegetables may be difficult for some clients to chew or digest. Wash fruits and vegetables well to remove any chemicals or pesticides.

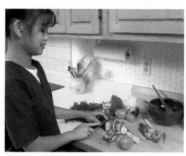

Fig. 6-8. *Many fruits and vegetables have the most nutrients when eaten uncooked and fresh.*

Preparing Mechanically Altered Diets

For soft, mechanical soft, or pureed diets, foods are prepared with blenders, food processors, or cutting utensils. Chopped foods are foods that have been cut up into very small pieces. When chopping food, use a sharp knife and a clean cutting board (separate boards for raw meat and for vegetables and other foods). Grinding breaks the foods up into even smaller pieces. Pureed foods are cooked and then ground very fine or strained. A little liquid is added to give them the consistency of baby food. Grinding and pureeing can be done in a blender or food processor. However, fruits and vegetables can also be pureed by pushing them through a colander with the back of a spoon.

All equipment used must be kept very clean to help prevent infection and illness. Take the blender or food processor apart after every use. Wash each piece that has come in contact with food in warm soapy water, and rinse thoroughly. Wash the cutting board after each use. This is especially important after chopping raw meat, poultry, and fish. Wash it with soap, or in the dishwasher, before using it again. Allow cutting board to air dry.

Changing the texture of food may make it lose its appeal. Season it according to the client's preferences to make it more appealing. Pureeing also causes nutrients to be lost, so vitamin supplements may be ordered. Constipation and dehydration are complications of a pureed diet. It is very important to follow directions exactly.

Preparing Nutritional Supplements

Illness and injury may call for nutritional supplements to be added into the client's diet. Certain medications also change the need for nutrients. Nutritional supplements may come in a powdered form or liquid form. Powdered supplements need to be mixed with a liquid before being taken; the care plan will include instructions on how much liquid to add.

When preparing supplements, make sure the supplement is mixed thoroughly. Make sure the client takes it at the ordered time. Clients who are ill, tired, or in pain may not have much of an appetite. It may take a long time for him to drink a large glass of a thick liquid. Be patient and encouraging. If a client does not want to drink the supplement, do not insist that he do so. However, do report this to your supervisor.

Guidelines: Safe Food Storage

G   Buy cold food last; get it home fast. After shopping, put away refrigerated foods first.

G   Keep it safe; refrigerate. Maintain refrigerator temperature between 36° and 40°F. Maintain freezer temperature at 0°F. Do not re-freeze items after they have been thawed. unfreeze

G   Use small containers that seal tightly. Foods cool more quickly when stored in smaller containers.

G   Never leave foods out for more than two hours.

G Tightly cover all foods. Store with enough room around them for air circulation. To prevent dry foods, such as cornmeal and flour, from becoming infested with insects, store these items in tightly sealed containers. Check dry storage areas periodically for signs of insects and rodents.

G Check the expiration dates on foods, especially perishables. Check the refrigerator frequently for spoiled foods. Discard any you find.

Cooking Safety

- Do not cook with long, loose sleeves that can catch on pot handles or catch fire.
- Turn pot handles toward the back of the stove to prevent tipping.
- Dry hands before using electrical appliances.
- Immediately clean any spills on the floor to prevent slipping.
- When lighting a gas stove or oven, light the match before turning on the gas. Be sure the match is extinguished and cool before throwing it away. Never use a match to light a self-lighting gas stove.
- Store potholders, dish towels, and other flammable kitchen items away from the stove.
- Stay in or near the kitchen when anything is cooking or baking. Never leave stove on and unattended.

Assisting a client with eating

Equipment: meal, eating utensils, clothing protector if appropriate, 1-2 napkins, wipes, or washcloths

1. Wash your hands.

2. Explain the procedure to the client, speaking clearly, slowly, and directly. Maintain face-to-face contact whenever possible.

3. If bed is adjustable, adjust bed height to where you will be able to sit at the client's eye level. Lock bed wheels.

4. Raise the head of the bed or use pillows to make sure that the client is in an upright sitting position (at a 90-degree angle).

5. Help the client wash her hands if client cannot do it on her own.

6. Help client put on clothing protector, if desired.

7. Sit facing client at the client's eye level (Fig. 6-9). Sit on the stronger side if the client has one-sided weakness.

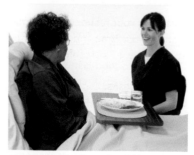

Fig. 6-9. The client should be sitting upright, and you should be sitting at her eye level.

8. Tell the client what foods make up the meal. Ask what client would like to eat first.

9. Check the temperature of the food. Test the temperature of the food by putting your hand over the dish to sense the heat. Do not touch food to test its temperature. If you think the food is too hot, do not blow on it to cool it. Offer other food to give it time to cool.

10. Offer the food in bite-sized pieces, telling the client the content of each bite of food offered. Alternate types of food offered, allowing for client's preferences. Do not feed all of one type before offering another type. Make sure the client's mouth is empty before offering the next bite of food or sip of drink.

11. Offer drinks throughout the meal. If you are holding the cup, touch it to the client's lips before you tip it. Give small, frequent sips. Use a straw or adaptive cup as necessary or as the client requests it.

12. Talk with the client throughout the meal. It makes mealtime more enjoyable. Do not rush the client.

13. Use washcloths, napkins, or wipes to wipe food from the client's mouth and hands as necessary during the meal. Wipe again at the end of the meal.

14. When the client is finished eating, remove the clothing protector if used. Remove the tray or dishes.

15. Assist the client to a comfortable position.

16. If you raised an adjustable bed, be sure to return it to its lowest position.

17. Wash your hands.

18. Document the client's intake, if required, and any observations. How did the client tolerate being upright for the meal? Did the client eat well? What foods did the client eat or not eat? Report any swallowing difficulties to your supervisor.

Managing Time and Money

Managing Time

Balancing your responsibilities means that you will need to learn ways to manage your time and energy efficiently. The following are ways to be sure your work schedule is as efficient as possible:

Distribute tasks. Look at the client care plan and your assignments. Note the assigned housekeeping tasks. Divide the tasks and schedule them for the week and the month. Make sure all your assignments can be completed in the time you have.

Prioritize tasks. Prioritizing your tasks is an important time and energy management skill. Think about the jobs you want to complete throughout the day. Which ones must be done immediately? Which ones must be done at a certain time? Which activities are not absolutely essential and could be put off? Spend time on activities that are most important first.

Simplify tasks. Learn to simplify your tasks. Take time to think about how you will go about doing a task. Try to eliminate a few steps but still get the same result.

Be realistic. You may not be able to get everything done, even if you plan carefully. When tasks take longer than you expected, or unexpected tasks need to be done, be realistic about what you can do. Do not be afraid to change your plan. Be flexible.

Many of the ideas for managing time on the job can be used to manage your personal time as well. The following are basic ways for managing time:

Plan ahead. Planning is the single best way to help you manage your time better.

Prioritize. Identify the most important things to get done. Do these first.

Make a schedule. Write out the hours of the day and fill in when you will do what.

Combine activities. Can you prepare tomorrow's dinner while the laundry is in the dryer? Work more efficiently when you can.

Get help. It is not reasonable for you to do everything. Do not be afraid to ask for help.

Work Plan

The client care plan and your assignments will tell you what tasks are required. You can develop your own work plan. This will allow you to finish all your assigned tasks as quickly and efficiently as possible. For each day or block of time you will spend in a home, list all the tasks you must complete. Then, prioritize them. Mark the most important as "1" and the next most important as "2," and so on. Finally, write out a schedule for the day, filling in the highest priority tasks first.

Remember to distribute tasks, so that you are not trying to do all the housecleaning in one afternoon and end up with no time to bathe or care for a client. Simplify tasks whenever possible to allow you to accomplish more.

Following an established work plan will also allow your clients and families to know what to expect of you. You may even want to discuss the plan with a client or family member as you are creating it or when it is finished. Some people appreciate knowing what will be happening in their homes at any given time.

Occasionally, you may be asked to do something that is not in the care plan or your assignments. There are several ways to handle requests that you must refuse. First, explain that you are only allowed to do tasks assigned in the care plan. Explain that nurses familiar with the client's condition give you your assignments. Emphasize that you would like to help, but you are limited to the tasks outlined in the care plan and your assignments. Contact your supervisor after explaining these points. Your supervisor may add the requested task to your assignments. Be sure to document the client's request and the actions you took to address it.

Client's Money

Different states and employers have different regulations and policies regarding healthcare employees handling clients' money. Find out from your employer whether you will be expected to handle clients' money. If you are not allowed to handle money, never agree to do so, even occasionally. You could get yourself and your employer in serious trouble.

Guidelines: Handling Clients' Money

G   Never use a client's money for your own needs, even if you plan to pay it back. This is considered stealing.

G   Estimate the amount of money you will need before requesting it. You may need to take things off your list or estimate the total bill as you go along in the store to stay within the money allotted.

G   Take checks, rather than cash, when possible. Have the client or family member fill out the name of the store. A signed check that is not made out is as good as cash.

G   Get a receipt for every purchase. This proves how much you spent and gives a record for you and the client.

G   Return receipts and change to client or family member immediately. Do not wait until the end of the day or week to settle up. Do it right away, while everything is fresh in your mind.

G   Keep a record of money you have spent. Follow your agency's policies for documenting money transactions. Write down how much you spent and where. Note any change returned to client. The better record you have, the smaller the chance of misunderstanding.

G Keep a client's cash separate from yours. If you must use the client's cash, do not put it in your own wallet. Keep it in a separate, safe place. Do the same with change. This will prevent confusion.

G Never offer money advice to a client. You should not even refer a client to others regarding their financial matters.

G Your clients' financial matters are confidential. Never discuss your clients' money matters with anyone.

VII.
Caring For Yourself

Continuing Education

Each state has slightly different requirements for maintaining certification. Be familiar with the requirements. Follow them exactly or you will not be able to keep working as an aide. Ask your instructor or employer for the requirements in your state. Know how many hours of in-service education are required per year. You also need to know how long an absence from working is allowed without retraining or recertification.

Some states do not have a registry for home health aides like the ones they maintain for certified nursing assistants (CNAs). If, for example, you have taken the certification exam for CNAs and are on the state registry, you may need to work a certain number of hours in a long-term care facility to remain on the registry. As a home health aide, ask your employer how best to maintain your certification.

The federal government requires that home health aides have 12 hours of continuing education each year. Some states may require more. "In-service" continuing education courses help you keep your knowledge and skills fresh. Classes may also provide you with more information about certain medical conditions, challenges that you face in working with clients, or regulation changes.

Your employer may be responsible for offering continuing education courses. However, you are responsible for attending and completing them. Specifically, you must do the following:

- Sign up for the course or find out where it is offered (Fig. 7-1).

- Attend all class sessions.

- Pay attention and complete all the class requirements.

- Make the most of your in-service programs. Participate!

- Keep original copies of all certificates and records of your successful attendance so you can prove you took the class.

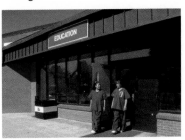

Fig. 7-1. *You may want to go outside the in-service programs offered by your employer to take some continuing education courses.*

Stress Management

Stress is the state of being frightened, excited, confused, in danger, or irritated. We usually think only bad things cause stress. However, positive situations cause stress, too. For example, getting married or having a baby are usually positive situations. But both can cause enormous stress because of the changes they bring to our lives.

You may be thrilled when you get a new job as a home health aide. But starting work may also cause you stress. You may be afraid of making mistakes, excited about earning money or helping people, or confused about how to perform your new duties. Learning how to recognize stress and what causes it is helpful. Then you can master a few simple techniques for relaxing and learn to manage stress.

A stressor is something that causes stress. Anything can be a stressor if it causes you stress. Some examples include:

- Divorce
- Marriage
- New baby
- Children growing up
- Children leaving home
- Feeling unprepared for a task
- Starting a new job
- Problems at work
- New responsibilities at work
- Losing a job
- Supervisors
- Co-workers
- Clients
- Illness
- Finances

Stress is not only an emotional response. It is also a physical response. When we experience stress, changes occur in our bodies. The endocrine system produces more of the hormone adrenaline. This can increase nervous system response, heart rate, respiratory rate, and blood pressure. This is why, in stressful situations, your heart beats fast, you breathe hard, and you feel warm or perspire.

Each of us has a different tolerance level for stress. In other words, what one person would find overwhelming may not bother another person. Your tolerance for stress depends on your personality, life experiences, and physical health.

Guidelines: Managing Stress

To manage stress in your life, develop healthy diet, exercise, and lifestyle habits:

G Eat nutritious foods.

G Exercise regularly.

G Get enough sleep.

G Drink only in moderation.

G Do not smoke.

G Find time at least a few times a week to do something relaxing.

Not managing stress can cause many problems. Some of these problems will affect how well you do your job. These are signs that you are not managing stress:

- Showing anger or being abusive toward clients
- Arguing with your supervisor about assignments
- Having poor relationships with co-workers and clients
- Complaining about your job and your responsibilities
- Feeling work-related burnout (burnout is a state of mental or physical exhaustion caused by stress)
- Feeling tired, even when you are rested
- Having trouble focusing on clients and procedures

Stress can seem overwhelming when you try to handle it by yourself. Often just talking about stress can help you manage it better. Sometimes another person can offer helpful suggestions. You may think of new ways to handle stress just by talking it through. Get help from one or more of the following when managing stress:

- Your supervisor or another member of the care team for work-related stress
- Your family
- Your friends
- Your place of worship

- Your doctor
- A local mental health agency
- Any phone hotline that deals with related problems (check the Internet or your local yellow pages)

It is not appropriate to turn to your clients or their family members about your personal or job-related stress. One of the best ways to manage is to develop a plan for managing stress. The plan can include things you will do every day and things to do in stressful situations. Before making a plan, you first need to answer these questions:

- What are the sources of stress in my life?
- When do I most often feel stress?
- What effects of stress do I see in my life?
- What can I change to decrease the stress I feel?
- What do I have to learn to cope with because I cannot change it?

When you have answered these questions, you will have a clearer picture of the challenges you face. Then you can try to come up with strategies for managing stress (Fig. 7-2).

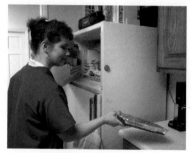

Fig. 7-2. *Keeping made-ahead meals in the refrigerator or freezer is a good way to eliminate stress.*

Your Career

Specialty training for HHAs is additional training to prepare an aide to care for clients with specific medical conditions. When a person becomes specialized, he or she learns as much as possible about that type of care in order to offer more advanced skills than those taught in basic training programs. The specialty-trained HHA has more education and more experience than other aides. He or she will be a better prepared caregiver. If you are interested in specialty training, consider the following:

- Choose a specialty that you seem to be more interested in than any other. Doing what you like to do every day is very important.
- Choose a specialty that your agency has the most referrals for, or that you know you can put to use in your particular area.

- Choose a program that is well-written and designed especially for your level of education and skills.

- Read as much as you can about this condition on your own.

- Discuss being assigned these types of clients with your supervisor.

- Talk to your clients who have this medical condition to gain some insight into their lives. Find out how they are affected from day to day.

After you are hired at an agency, there may be times you will need to make a complaint or voice a concern about some part of your job. Do not be afraid to do this, but do it carefully.

Think about the problem. Some major problems must be reported right away. For example, if a client, family member, or coworker threatens you, report this to your supervisor immediately. Other problems may work themselves out in time. If a new client seems rude, it is possible that he or she feels uncomfortable with new people or does not understand your role. You may want to wait several days or weeks to see if things improve before making a complaint. Know which problems should be reported immediately to your supervisor.

Plan what you will say. Think through and even write out what you will say to your supervisor. This will help you present your complaint clearly and completely.

Do not get emotional. Some situations may be very upsetting. However, you will be more effective in communicating and problem-solving if you can keep your emotions out of it. Share your feelings about a situation— whether you are mad, hurt, or annoyed—with a friend. Tell your supervisor the facts.

Do not hesitate to communicate situations that you feel are important or that may put you or a client at risk. One common problem in home care is aides not reporting when they feel unsafe at a particular client's home. In this case, not complaining can prove dangerous for you and the client. Always report to your supervisor any situation in which you feel you or the client is at risk of harm, even if the situation involves the client's family or friends.

If you decide to change jobs, be responsible. Always give your employer at least two weeks' written notice that you will be leaving. Otherwise, assignments may be left uncovered, or other aides may have to work more until the agency fills your spot. In addition, future employers may talk with past supervisors. People who change jobs too often or who do not give notice before leaving are less likely to be hired.

Look back over all you have learned in this program. Your work as a home health aide is very important. Every day may be different and challenging. In a hundred ways every week you will offer help that only a caring person like you can provide.

Do not forget to value the work you have chosen to do. It is important. For your clients, your work can mean the difference between living at home and living in an institution. It can mean living with independence and dignity versus living without. The difference you make is sometimes life versus death. Look in the face of each of your clients and know that you are doing important work. Look in a mirror when you get home and be proud of how you make your living.

An important life skill is being able to reflect on how you spend your time. Learn ways to fully appreciate that what you do has great meaning. Few jobs have the challenges and rewards of home health care. Congratulate yourself for choosing a path that includes helping others along the way.

Abbreviations

ā	before
ABR	absolute bedrest
ac, a.c.	before meals
ADL	activities of daily living
AIDS	acquired immune deficiency syndrome
am, AM	morning, before noon
amb	ambulate, ambulatory
amt	amount
ap	apical
as tol	as tolerated
ax.	axillary (armpit)
b.i.d., BID	two times a day
BM	bowel movement
BP, B/P	blood pressure
BPM	beats per minute
BRP	bathroom privileges
c̄	with
C	Centigrade
cath.	catheter
CBC	complete blood count
CBR	complete bedrest
CDC	Centers for Disease Control
C. diff	*clostridium difficile*
CHF	congestive heart failure
c/o	complains of

COPD	chronic obstructive pulmonary disease
CPR	cardiopulmonary resuscitation
CVA	cerebrovascular accident, stroke
DNR	do not resuscitate
DON	director of nursing
Dx, dx	diagnosis
EMS	emergency medical services
F	Fahrenheit or female
FF	force fluids
ft	foot
F/U, f/u	follow-up
FWB	full weight bearing
h, hr, hr.	hour
H_2O	water
H/A, HA	headache
HBV	hepatitis B virus
HHA	home health aide
HIPAA	Health Insurance Portability and Accountability Act
HIV	human immunodeficiency virus
HOB	head of bed
ht	height
HTN	hypertension
hyper	above normal, too fast, rapid
hypo	low, less than normal

I&O	intake and output
inc	incontinent
isol	isolation
IV, I.V.	intravenous (within a vein)
lab	laboratory
lb.	pound
LTC	long-term care
meds	medications
mL	milliliter
mmHg	millimeters of mercury
MRSA	methicillin-resistant *Staphylococcus aureus*
N/A	not applicable
NKA	no known allergies
NPO	nothing by mouth
NVD	nausea, vomiting and diarrhea
NWB	non-weight bearing
O_2	oxygen
OBRA	Omnibus Budget Reconciliation Act
OOB	out of bed
oz	ounce
$\bar{p}$	after
peri care	perineal care
per os, PO	by mouth
PPE	personal protective equipment
p.r.n., prn	when necessary
PVD	peripheral vascular disease
PWB	partial weight bearing
$\bar{q}$	every
q2h	every two hours
q3h	every three hours
q4h	every four hours
R	respirations, rectal
rehab	rehabilitation
RF	restrict fluids
R.I.C.E.	rest, ice, compression, elevation
RN	registered nurse
R/O	rule out
ROM	range of motion
$\bar{s}$	without
SOB	shortness of breath
spec.	specimen
stat	immediately
std. prec.	Standard Precautions
T., temp	temperature
TB	tuberculosis
t.i.d., TID	three times a day
TPR	temperature, pulse, and respiration
UTI	urinary tract infection
VS, vs	vital signs
w/c, W/C	wheelchair
wt.	weight

Glossary

abuse: purposely causing physical, mental, or emotional pain or injury to someone.

acquired immune deficiency syndrome (AIDS): disease caused by the human immunodeficiency virus (HIV) in which the body's immune system is weakened and unable to fight infection.

active neglect: purposely harming a person by failing to provide needed care.

activities of daily living (ADLs): personal daily care tasks, such as bathing, dressing, caring for teeth and hair, toileting, eating and drinking, walking, and transferring.

agitation: being excited, restless, or troubled.

Alzheimer's disease (AD): progressive, incurable disease that causes tangled nerve fibers and protein deposits to form in the brain, which eventually cause dementia.

ambulation: walking.

ambulatory: capable of walking.

angina pectoris: the medical term for chest pain, pressure, or discomfort.

anorexia: an eating disorder in which a person does not eat or exercises excessively to lose weight.

antimicrobial: capable of destroying or resisting pathogens.

anxiety: uneasiness or fear, often about a situation or condition.

arthritis: a general term that refers to inflammation of the joints that causes stiffness, pain, and decreased mobility.

aspiration: the inhalation of food, fluid, or foreign material into the lungs; can cause pneumonia or death.

asthma: a chronic inflammatory disease that causes difficulty breathing, coughing and wheezing.

atrophy: the wasting away, decreasing in size, and weakening of muscles from lack of use.

bloodborne pathogens: microorganisms found in human blood, body fluids, draining wounds, and mucous membranes that can cause infection and disease in humans.

body mechanics: the way the parts of the body work together whenever a person moves.

bronchitis: an irritation and inflammation of the lining of the bronchi.

cardiopulmonary resuscitation (CPR): medical procedures used when a person's heart or lungs have stopped working.

catheter: a thin tube inserted into the body used to drain fluids or inject fluids.

cerebrovascular accident (CVA): a condition that occurs when blood supply to a part of the brain is cut off suddenly by a clot or a ruptured blood vessel; also called a stroke.

chronic: long-term or long-lasting.

chronic obstructive pulmonary disorder (COPD): a chronic lung disease that cannot be cured; causes difficulty breathing.

cognitive: related to thinking and learning.

colostomy: surgically-created diversion of stool or feces to an artificial opening through the abdomen; stool will generally be semi-solid.

combustion: the process of burning.

compassionate: caring, concerned, considerate, empathetic, and understanding.

confidentiality: the legal and ethical principle of keeping information private.

congestive heart failure (CHF): a condition in which the heart is no longer able to pump effectively; blood backs up into the heart instead of circulating.

conscientious: guided by a sense of right and wrong; having principles.

constipation: the inability to eliminate stool, or the difficult elimination of a hard, dry stool.

constrict: to narrow.

contracture: the permanent and often painful stiffening of a joint and muscle.

culture: a system of learned behaviors, practiced by a group of people, that are considered to be the tradition of that people and are passed on from one generation to the next.

cyanotic: skin that is pale, blue, or gray.

dangle: to sit up with the feet over the side of the bed in order to regain balance.

dehydration: a condition that results from inadequate fluid in the body.

dementia: a general term that refers to a serious loss of mental abilities, such as thinking, remembering, reasoning, and communicating.

depression: a serious mental illness that may cause intense mental, emotional, and physical pain and disability.

diabetes: a condition in which the pancreas does not produce enough or does not properly use insulin; causes problems with circulation and can damage vital organs.

diabetic ketoacidosis (DKA): complication of diabetes that is caused by having too little insulin; also called hyperglycemia.

diarrhea: frequent elimination of liquid or semi-liquid feces.

diastolic: second measurement of blood pressure; phase when the heart relaxes or rests.

digestion: the process of preparing food physically and chemically so that it can be absorbed into the cells.

dilate: to widen.

direct contact: touching an infected person or his secretions.

disorientation: confusion about person, place, or time.

draw sheet: an extra sheet placed on top of a bottom sheet to help with turning, lifting or moving clients.

dysphagia: difficulty swallowing.

dyspnea: difficulty breathing.

elimination: the process of expelling solid wastes made up of the waste products of food that are not absorbed into the cells.

emesis: the act of vomiting, or ejecting stomach contents through the mouth.

emotional lability: laughing or crying without any reason, or when it is inappropriate.

epilepsy: an illness of the brain that causes seizures.

ethics: the knowledge of right and wrong.

exposure control plan: plan designed to eliminate or reduce employee exposure to infectious material.

expressive aphasia: inability to speak or speak clearly.

first aid: emergency care given immediately to an injured person.

flammable: easily ignited and capable of burning quickly.

fluid balance: taking in and eliminating equal amounts of fluid.

foot drop: a weakness of muscles in the feet and ankles that causes problems with the ability to flex the ankles and walk normally.

fracture: a broken bone.

gait belt: a belt made of canvas or other heavy material used to assist people who are who are weak, unsteady, or uncoordinated; also called a transfer belt.

gastroesophageal reflux disease (GERD): a chronic condition in which the liquid contents of the stomach back up into the esophagus; causes bleeding or ulcers and difficulty swallowing.

glands: structures that produce substances in the body.

glaucoma: a condition in which the fluid inside the eyeball is unable to drain; increased pressure inside the eye causes damage that often leads to blindness.

hand antisepsis: washing hands with water and soap or other detergents that contain an antiseptic agent.

hand hygiene: washing hands with either plain or antiseptic soap and water and using alcohol-based hand rubs.

health maintenance organizations (HMOs): a method of health insurance in which a person has to use a particular doctor or group of doctors except in case of emergency.

hemiparesis: weakness on one side of the body.

hemiplegia: paralysis on one side of the body.

hepatitis: inflammation of the liver caused by infection.

HIV: stands for human immunodeficiency virus, the virus that can cause AIDS.

homeostasis: the condition in which all of the body's systems are working their best.

hormones: chemical substances created by the body that control numerous body functions.

hygiene: practices used to keep bodies clean and healthy.

hypertension: high blood pressure.

incident report: a report that must be completed when an accident or other unexpected event occurs during a visit.

incontinence: the inability to control the bladder or bowels.

indirect contact: touching something contaminated by an infected person.

infection control: measures practiced in healthcare facilities and other settings to prevent and control the spread of disease.

infectious: contagious.

insulin reaction: complication of diabetes that can result from either too much insulin or too little food; also known as hypoglycemia.

intake: the fluid a person consumes; also called input.

intravenous (IV): into a vein.

laws: rules set by the government to help people live peacefully together and to ensure order and safety.

liability: a legal term that means someone can be held responsible for harming someone else.

Medicaid: a medical assistance program for low-income people.

medical asepsis: the process of removing pathogens, or the state of being free of pathogens.

Medicare: a federal health insurance program for people who are 65 or older, are disabled, or are ill and cannot work.

metabolism: physical and chemical processes by which substances are produced or broken down into energy or products for use by the body.

microorganism: a living thing or organism that is so small that it can be seen only through a microscope; also called a microbe.

mucous membranes: the membranes that line body cavities, such as the mouth, nose, eyes, rectum, or genitals.

multiple sclerosis (MS): a progressive disease of the nervous system in which the protective covering for the nerves, spinal cord, and white matter of the brain breaks down over time; without this covering, nerves cannot send messages to and from the brain in a normal way.

myocardial infarction (MI): a condition that occurs when the heart muscle does not receive enough oxygen because blood vessels are blocked; also called a heart attack.

neglect: harming a person physically, mentally, or emotionally by failing to provide needed care.

neuropathy: numbness, tingling, and pain in the feet and legs.

nonverbal communication: communicating without using words.

Occupational Safety and Health Administration (OSHA): a federal government agency that makes rules to protect workers from hazards on the job.

orthotic device: a device that helps support and align a limb and improve its functioning and helps prevent or correct deformities.

osteoporosis: a disease that causes bones to become porous and brittle.

ostomy: a surgically-created opening from an area inside the body to the outside.

output: all fluid that is eliminated from the body; includes fluid in urine, feces, vomitus, perspiration, and moisture in the air that is exhaled.

oxygen therapy: the administration of oxygen to increase the supply of oxygen to the lungs.

palliative care: care that focuses on the comfort and dignity of the person, rather than on curing him or her.

passive neglect: unintentionally harming a person physically, mentally, or emotionally by failing to provide needed care.

pathogen: disease-causing microorganism.

perineal care: care of the genital and anal area.

perseveration: repeating words, phrases, questions, or actions.

personal protective equipment (PPE): equipment that helps protect employees from serious workplace injuries or illnesses resulting from contact with workplace hazards.

phobia: an intense form of anxiety or fear.

physical abuse: any treatment, intentional or not, that causes harm to a person's body; includes slapping, bruising, cutting, burning, physically restraining, pushing, shoving, or rough handling.

policy: a course of action that should be taken every time a certain situation occurs.

preferred provider organizations (PPOs): a network of providers that contract to provide health services to a group of people.

pressure sore: a serious wound resulting from skin breakdown; also known as decubitus ulcer, pressure ulcer, or bed sore.

procedure: a method, or way, of doing something.

prosthesis: a device that replaces a body part that is missing or deformed because of an accident, injury, illness, or birth defect; used to improve a person's ability to function and/or his appearance.

psychological abuse: any behavior that causes a person to feel threatened, fearful, intimidated, or humiliated in any way.

psychosocial needs: needs having to do with social interaction, emotions, intellect, and spirituality.

range of motion (ROM) exercises: exercises that put a joint through its full arc of motion.

receptive aphasia: inability to understand spoken or written words.

respiration: the process of breathing air into the lungs and exhaling air out of the lungs.

schizophrenia: a brain disorder that affects a person's ability to think and communicate clearly, as well as manage emotions, make decisions, and understand reality.

scope of practice: defines the things that healthcare providers are legally allowed to do and how to do them correctly.

sexual abuse: forcing a person to perform or participate in sexual acts against his or her will; includes unwanted touching, exposing oneself, and sharing pornographic material.

sexually transmitted diseases (STDs): diseases caused by sexual contact with an infected person; also called venereal diseases.

sexually transmitted infections (STIs): infections caused by sexual contact with an infected person; a person may be infected, and may potentially infect others, without showing signs of the disease.

sharps: needles or other sharp objects.

shearing: rubbing or friction that results from the skin moving one way and the bone underneath it remaining fixed or moving in the opposite direction.

specimen: a sample that is used for analysis in order to try to make a diagnosis.

sputum: the fluid a person coughs up from the lungs.

Standard Precautions: a method of infection control in which all blood, body fluids, non-intact skin, and mucous membranes are treated as if they were infected with an infectious disease.

stoma: an artificial opening in the body.

sundowning: becoming restless and agitated in the late afternoon, evening, or night.

systolic: first measurement of blood pressure; phase when the heart is at work, contracting and pushing the blood from the left ventricle of the heart.

tactful: being able to understand what is proper and appropriate when dealing with others; being able to speak and act without offending others.

terminal illness: a disease or condition that will eventually cause death.

transfer belt: a belt made of canvas or other heavy material, used to assist people who are weak, unsteady, or uncoordinated; also called a gait belt.

tuberculosis (TB): an airborne disease that affects the lungs; causes coughing, trouble breathing, fever, weight loss, and fatigue.

tumor: a group of abnormally growing cells.

validating: giving value to or approving.

verbal abuse: the use of language—spoken or written—that threatens, embarrasses, or insults a person.

Index

Names/Numbers You Should Know

Abuse Hotline

Alzheimer's Association (local)

Area Agency on Aging

Church/Spiritual Advisor

Dietitian

Errand Service

Family Members

Fire Department

HHA Agency

Hospice

Meals on Wheels

Medical Supply Company

Natural Disaster Information Line

Pharmacist

Physician

Poison Control Center

Police Department (Non-Emergency)

Public Transportation

Senior Citizens' Center

Supervisor

Transportation Services

Other Resources: